Health Education Teaching Ideas:

SECONDARY

Richard Loya, *Editor*

**Association for the Advancement
of Health Education**

an association of the

**American Alliance for
Health, Physical Education,
Recreation and Dance**

ISBN 0-83314-238-4

Purposes of the American Alliance For Health, Physical Education, Recreation and Dance

The American Alliance is an educational organization, structured for the purposes of supporting, encouraging, and providing assistance to member groups and their personnel throughout the nation as they seek to initiate, develop, and conduct programs in health, leisure, and movement-related activities for the enrichment of human life.

Alliance objectives include:

1. Professional growth and development—to support, encourage, and provide guidance in the development and conduct of programs in health, leisure, and movement-related activities which are based on the needs, interests, and inherent capacities of the individual in today's society.

2. Communication—to facilitate public and professional understanding and appreciation of the importance and value of health, leisure, and movement-related activities as they contribute toward human well-being.

3. Research—to encourage and facilitate research which will enrich the depth and scope of health, leisure, and movement-related activities; and to disseminate the findings to the profession and other interested and concerned publics.

4. Standards and guidelines—to further the continuous development and evaluation of standards within the profession for personnel and programs in health, leisure, and movement-related activities.

5. Public affairs—to coordinate and administer a planned program of professional, public, and governmental relations that will improve education in areas of health, leisure, and movement-related activities.

6. To conduct such other activities as shall be approved by the Board of Governors and the Alliance Assembly, provided that the Alliance shall not engage in any activity which would be inconsistent with the status of an educational and charitable organization as defined in Section 501(c) (3) of the Internal Revenue Code of 1954 or any successor provision thereto, and none of the said purposes shall at any time be deemed or construed to be purposes other than the public benefit purposes and objectives consistent with such educational and charitable status.   *Bylaws, Article III*

Foreword

Where is *health* taught at the secondary level? In the elementary school it is usually taught by the elementary teacher along with twenty or so other subjects. In the junior and senior high schools it can be found in many places: health classes; science classes; family living classes; social science classes; home economics classes; and drivers' education classes. In the school district where I taught, it was found in one high school in a class entitled "State Requirements." This unique class included all the "loose end" topics that were required by the State of California to be covered before high school graduation.

Wherever health is taught in the schools, the ultimate success with students is not determined by the title of the class or placement within the curriculum. It is largely dependent upon the quality of the teaching. *Health* can be the most exciting, interesting, and meaningful class in the high school curriculum. Dedicated, energetic, caring teachers do make a difference. Talented teachers can motivate and positively affect the lives of the most gifted students as well as the ones with special problems. This book, *Health Education Teaching Ideas: Secondary,* is for those teachers. It includes innovative teaching strategies that are practical and appropriate in the secondary classroom. The original articles appeared in the "Teaching Ideas" column of *Health Education* and were compiled by a high school health teacher. This book should be a useful and exciting addition to the library of any instructor responsible for health education at the junior and senior high school levels.

Kathleen Middleton, *Director*
School Health Programs
National Center for Health Education
and Contributing Editor to
"Teaching Ideas" column of
Health Education

CONTENTS

Foreword, *Kathleen Middleton*

Focus on Process

Focus on Content

Addictive Behaviors

Aging

Consumer Health

Death and Dying

Environmental Health

Family Life

Focus on Process

Stress on Reading

ELAINE HALS is a teacher of health education at South Shore High School, Brooklyn, New York 11236.

In the last few years large cities throughout the United States have begun to put pressure on school districts to stress the "three R's"—more reading, more math, and more writing. In New York City, where I teach, all of the principals have been instructed to increase the number of periods per week devoted to reading and other basics in the elementary schools. The high schools have been instructed that all subject areas give reading and written homework several times weekly, and that course curriculum should stress the basics. Employers have also been pressuring the schools to improve the reading ability of their graduates. The push is now on to raise the basic skills level of today's youth.

How does this push for basics affect us as health educators? Do we regress to predominantly cognitive teaching? Do we return to stressing facts, and only those things that can be read, written, and tested? About ten years ago health educators began to realize the importance of humanistic values and behavior modification that could be accomplished in health teaching. Our field has seen positive changes, and we have shifted our emphasis into the affective domain. Health education has truly become learning for living—examination of values, decision making, and behavioral alternatives. If we help young people become better, healthier, and more aware, but do not help them to read better, are we in line with the educational goals of the country? Should we be? The pendulum has swung back to pre-1960s education. Should we as health educators re-evaluate our goals, and fall in line with other subject areas? Reading and writing are important; I do not mean to demean their significance. Young people entering the job market must have basic skills in order to survive.

Because both affective and cognitive education are valuable, I feel that we as health educators must combine them in our teaching. Following you will find a few suggestions.

1. Help students to explore new and controversial health issues by having them read and evaluate current newspaper and magazine articles on various subjects—laetrile, cloning, test tube babies, food additives, new drugs, disease cures.

2. Have students keep a written log (to be checked by the teacher periodically) of feelings about the class, their daily decisions, new material learned, or anything the teacher feels is relevant to the class and the students.

3. Have students keep their own vocabulary list of new words learned in class or from text, pamphlets or other reading sources.

4. Have students write letters requesting information, pamphlets, interviews.

5. Offer reading lists of novels, magazines, etc. for outside projects or just additional information.

6. Give students controversial problems for homework and have them write answers that can later be discussed in class and even made into role playing situations.

> Your parents catch you and your friends smoking grass in your room, what would you do?
> You are caught cheating on an exam and the teacher wants to see your parents.

> You find that you have venereal disease—your boy or girl friend may have it, too—what do you do?
> Do the terminally ill have the right to know they are dying?
> You know something that could get your best friend in trouble. You feel what this person did was wrong. You are going to be questioned about the situation. What will you do?

7. Use pamphlets and current publications instead of, or in addition to, text books.

8. Divide class into groups. Have each group research and investigate different aspects of a subject and teach the class.

9. Creative projects that combine reading and writing with other disciplines such as art, photography, music.

10. Have class construct interviews or surveys, then have students survey or interview selected individuals and evaluate results.

Cognitive and affective can be made to work well together. We do not have to forsake our humanistic, affective approach to health education in order to help our students read and write better. Instead of changing the educational goals we have for our students, we should just add one more—a better knowledge of the basics and how they can help our students live better, healthier lives.

Affective Evaluation Techniques in School Health Education

Mary S. Sutherland is associate professor in the Department of Human Studies at Florida State University, Tallahassee, Florida 32306.

Affective measures of evaluation attempt to indicate how a person feels about an idea or subject. Krothwohl[1] in designing the affective taxonomy proposed various degrees of internalization of values, ranging through awareness, willingness to receive, controlled attention, acquiescence in responding, willingness to respond, satisfaction in response, acceptance of value, preference for a value, commitment, conceptualization of a value, preference for a value system, a generalized set, and finally characterization of a particular value. The continuum of affective responses is further divided into five main categories of internalization: receiving, responding, valuing, organization, and characterization.

The quote, "You are a product of every moment you have lived until today," will in part determine responses to any affective questions asked of individuals. Considering the varied backgrounds and experiences within any school population, effective measurement and evaluation in the affective domain can be difficult. Many individuals unfamiliar with the affective domain or attitudinal measurement, have opined that the schools are teaching specific teacher held values, instead of the valuing process. These individuals should be introduced to the above information as well as to the decision-making process, such as that popularized by Simon and used by many health educators in the classroom. Numerous methodologies have been proposed for the measurement of attitudes, some valid and reliable, others not. A sample listing follows of possible affective measurement techniques and appropriate examples of their application in health education. The techniques are presented in no particular order.

Thurston Attitude Scales

This is an equal-appearing-interval procedure that represents various strengths of feelings toward a given statement, objective, or situation. Each statement is weighted by judges to reflect degrees of feelings. The design of the instrument, in order to construct a valid and reliable scale, can be a time consuming process.

Directions: X = Disagree   L = Agree
Using these symbols on the exercise below, please indicate how you personally stand on the issues listed.

_____ 1. (1.5) Drug abusers are only hurting themselves.

_____ 2. (2.0) A poor self concept may lead to drug abuse.

_____ 3. (2.5) Inability to make decisions based on the consequences of the desired behavior may lead to drug abuse.

Likert Scale

One of the most widely used techniques is the Likert Scale. Statements are constructed with responses on a five point continuum of strongly agree, agree, undecided, disagree, and strongly disagree. The testee selects the answer that best describes his/her reaction to the situation.

Directions: Please circle your response to the following statements. Strongly agree = SA; Agree = A; Undecided = U; Disagree = D; Strongly disagree = SD.

1. People abuse drugs when they possess a poor self concept.
   SA   A   U   D   SD
2. Excessive peer pressure may cause a person to abuse drugs.
   SA   A   U   D   SD
3. Some drugs may serve a useful purpose.
   SA   A   U   D   SD

Sort

Individuals are given sets of cards containing statements, traits, or pictures. They are then requested to sort these into piles according to their relative applicability, i.e. *most like me* to *least like me*. An example in a health course would be to distribute pictures of teenagers participating in various activities, and then to have the students indicate which are most and least applicable.

Forced Choice

Individuals are encouraged to select one of several given responses as an expression of their attitudes—similar to the interview technique described below, except that individuals are not asked specific questions.

Directions: Please indicate if you would choose the first option presented in the question, or the second.

1	2	Statements
_____	_____	1. I would rather be alone or with my friends.
_____	_____	2. I prefer to work individually or within small groups.
_____	_____	3. I would rather go to a movie or take a drive in the country.

Interview

The interview is a face-to-face encounter, in which the interviewer asks the testee specific questions. Little deviation from the questionnaire is allowed, except to clarify ambiguous answers.

1. Should drug abusers be encouraged to seek treatment or not to seek treatment?
2. Should drug abusers be encouraged to improve their self concepts, or maintain their present self concepts?
3. Should drug abusers improve decision-making processes, or continue present decision-making practices?

Rating Scales

Rating scales are similar to the Likert Scale, except that instead of using a standard set of options, specific adjective/verb describers are utilized:

Directions: Circle your response about drug abuses on the continuum

DRUG ABUSERS	Possess no self concept.	Possess a poor self concept.	Possess a good self concept.
DRUG ABUSERS	Find it very difficult to communicate.	Find it difficult to communicate.	Find it easy to communicate.
DRUG ABUSERS	Find it very difficult to make a decision.	Find it difficult to make a decision.	Find it easy to make a decision.

Rating scales can be developed with three to seven responses, using describers or single adjectives. The final form should depend on the particular purpose for the utilization of the instrument.

Semantic Differential

In this instrument concepts are measured in terms of evaluation (good-bad), potency (weak-strong), and activity (fast-slow). The respondent checks his response on the scale; the evaluation process assists in distinguishing differences between concepts and individual responses.

Directions: Place an X on the scale to indicate your feelings about each statement below.

ABUSING DRUGS IS:

Good	____	____	____	____	____	Bad
Foolish	____	____	____	____	____	Wise
Beneficial	____	____	____	____	____	Harmful

DRUGS CAN BE:

Good	____	____	____	____	____	Bad
Foolish	____	____	____	____	____	Wise
Beneficial	____	____	____	____	____	Harmful

Open-ended Questions

The open-ended question calls for the respondent to answer by writing statements which reflect an attitude, belief, activity or value. It can assist in measuring attitude structure and socialization.

1. Drug abusers should be encouraged to _____
_____ .
2. Drug abuse is _____
_____ .
3. A positive self concept is _____ .

Projected Techniques

Projected techniques are designed to reveal information about a person's deeper levels of feelings, and his reactions to a phenomenon via pictures. Generally given are the beginning, middle, and ending of a situation related to the pictures, from which the testee must be able to write a complete story.

Projected Behavior

Students are placed in a hypothetical situation and are requested to determine how they would behave under those circumstances.

Bob and Dan are friends of long standing. Bob tries to interest Dan in smoking a joint. Dan should:
a. Smoke the joint.
b. Refuse to take the joint.
c. Take the joint and later throw it away.
d. Take the joint and later smoke it in private.

Additional techniques to be utilized include check lists and ranking sheets, classroom teacher observations, anecdotal records (summaries of attitudes/behavior by the school staff), time sampling (what happened when), sociograms, social distance scales, guess-who questionnaires, and autobiographical sketches.

In contrasting and comparing the various methods utilized for attitude assessment, it is most necessary to establish a set and a setting for instrument utilization. Each of the abovementioned instruments can serve a valid and reliable purpose if applied correctly in the situation for which it was designed.

Affective measurement and evaluation techniques could be used for health instruction in many ways.

1. *To determine student behavioral information to assist in the removal of barriers to the efficient/effective functioning of the classroom educational process.* Specifically with the so-called behavioral problem student, cumulative records are useful to reinforce comments from anecdotal records and previous teacher time sample studies. A sociogram exercise conducted within the class determines the problem student's social status within his peer group; but more importantly, teachers and administrators should observe student attitude and behaviors for true indicators of causes of specific problems. In addition, a clue to behavioral problems is gained from a problem checklist and the professional psychological technique of a Q Sort described above. However, in the final analysis, the teacher must usually sit down with the problem student and communicate directly. The proper leading questions should serve to flush out information related to the true causes of the problem—is it lack of interest and motivation, poor self-concept, poor communication skills, uncomfortable environment or what? The causes of poor behavior can usually be determined by using one or a combination of affective techniques. An appropriate plan of action should be developed by the student, to change his behavior to a more acceptable level for the classroom.

2. *Health Instruction.* Many of these attitudinal devices find their best use in the area of classroom instruction. A Thurstone attitude scale takes considerable time to develop and field-test, but indicates most clearly differing degrees of feelings toward a topic or statement. If the health educator has time to computer-score results, the Likert scales are most useful to compare differences in attitudes. A modified version of the

Likert suits small group discussion activities, as do rating scales, ranking scales, checklists, open-ended sentences, projected behavior techniques and closed sentences directed towards specific behavioral objectives. Activities should be deliberately processed, so that principles of communication, self-concept and decision-making may be applied to specific health content areas. The abovementioned techniques are marvelous ways in which the class and teacher can get to know and appreciate each other, as well as marvelous stepping stones to effective teaching/learning. In summary, an affective technique can be a learning activity, a way of reinforcing and applying specific content covered, and lastly, can be one of many techniques to evaluate an effective health education program.

3. *Attitude Measurement.* The methods and techniques described above measure changing attitudes, both short term and long term. Instruments most helpful in measuring attitudes include Thurstone scales, Likert scales, rating scales, behavioral projected techniques, and behavioral practices checklists. Great attention should be paid to fakability, semantics, and criterion inadequacy. Is the student merely feeding to the teacher what the teacher wants to hear? Do the terms of questions and statements mean the same thing to the tester and the testee? Does the test really measure what it is supposed to?

4. *Evaluation of Classroom Learning.* Attitudinal devices such as open-ended sentences serve to indicate both teacher effectiveness or learning effectiveness. Specific open-ended questions might include:

A. Today I learned _____ .

B. Today I relearned _____ .

C. Today, I wish _____ .

In this manner the health educator gains insight into the student's evaluation of what is going on in the classroom:

In the final analysis, the setting as related to health education should determine the type of instrument used to obtain the most valid and reliable information possible for the most efficient/effective use of time and money for all concerned parties and purposes.

---

[1]J. Stanley and K. Hopkins. *Educational and psychological measurement and evaluation.* Englewood Cliffs, New Jersey, 1977, 229.

Five Cures for Dull Health Curriculums

LOREN B. BENSLEY, JR., is professor of health education, Central Michigan University, Mt. Pleasant, Michigan 48858.

The health education philosophies, concepts, and attitudes of the past are present in many of today's curriculums and are breeding irrelevant, dull, meaningless, distasteful classes in health education.

We are in a time of educational revolutions. Students are questioning our systems, curriculums, teacher qualifications, and pedagogy. They find themselves trapped in an educational system intent on turning them into mechanical robots; irrelevant curriculums combined with poor teachers are forced on them. Fortunately, educational systems are trying to change, but much of the change is no more than an attempt to refine the existing machinery, making it ever more efficient in pursuit of obsolete goals. Alvin Toffler, in his book *Future Shock,* suggests that "instead of assuming that every subject taught today is taught for a reason [we] should begin from the reverse premise: nothing should be included in a required curriculum unless it can be strongly justified in terms of the future. If this means scrapping a substantial part of the formal curriculum, so be it." [1]

Today millions of students are forced through health classes and exposed to meaningless experiences which will in no way result in favorable health behavior.

What evidence do we have to show the public that we are accomplishing our objectives? Will a student be a healthier citizen because of a course in health education?

It is time that we in health education produce results, not a collection of meaningless philosophical statements and purposes. In order to produce results two components must be integrated: a relevant curriculum and a creative and committed health educator. When these two components are plugged into each other, there will be generated electricity, excitement, enthusiasm, and vibrations in the student to turn him on to health learning. Only when the curriculum and the teacher are united will there be an illumination of the student. One without the other will result in total darkness. Unfortunately, much of our school health education has not had the proper electrical engineering to illuminate proper health attitudes and behaviors of our students.

Health education may not be as bleak as the author has presented it. Recent years have brought new insights and encouragement to curriculum development in health education. Approximately ten years ago we had a national school health education study. From this was devised a sophisticated curriculum based on the conceptual approach. About four years ago, the state of Connecticut did a comprehensive study on the health needs and interests of school children. Their document titled "Teach Us What We Want To Know" is extremely valuable in the hands of the health educator. Most of us are familiar with the efforts of New York State in designing a curriculum for their public schools. Their most recent adventure in computerized individualized instruction is certainly encouraging. The State of Michigan is presently developing a curriculum K through 14 in health education. From the most recent drug abuse crisis have resulted some excellent curriculums in this specific subject matter.

Health in Three Grades Only

These new efforts are encouraging; however, the relevance of some of the products that have been prepared are questionable. Take, for example, the school health education study curriculum produced by the 3M Company. The curriculum is so sophisticated and so complicated that 90% of our classroom teachers in Michigan are discouraged from using it. It cannot be said that it isn't a good piece of work; it is in fact a product of excellence. Unfortunately, it's not realistic. This author questions how realistic the K-12 concept is without trained health educators or health coordinators. Wouldn't it be better in health education to isolate three grade levels where health could be emphasized? I suggest that possibly health education be taught in the fourth, seventh, and eleventh grades.

I selected these grade levels because these are the ages where we can help our students develop desirable health behaviors. The nine-year-old has a keen interest in his body as well as in health in general. He shows excitement in learning about the function of his total being. The seventh-grader, on the other hand, is at the critical age in developing positive health behaviors. At age 12 he is confronted with decisions about whether or not he should smoke or experiment with alcohol or drugs. At this age secondary sex characteristics develop, which create a variety of physical and mental problems. The eleventh-grade student has reached the age of sophistication and needs information that will guide his behavior as an adult. He is now a health consumer and soon will be faced with health insurance decisions as well as a multitude of other alternatives. We must also realize that within three years at least half of the girls will be married.

New Names Can Be Magic

In a typical health course in the public schools, units have such titles as Mental Health, First Aid, Sex Education, Alcohol, Tobacco, Drugs and Narcotics, etc. The titles of these units themselves are enough

5

to turn the students off to health. We were plagued for years with the term "hygiene" until the 1920s, when Sally Lucas Jean came up with the term "health education," indicating the change from hygiene teaching to behavior modification. I think the time has arrived when we, as health educators, can be more creative and original in making the appearance of our curriculum exciting to the learner. Just a change in titles of the units may turn a student on to health learning rather than turn him off from what he would anticipate as a dreadful experience. For instance, instead of calling a unit First Aid, why not title it Emergency Medical Care? Sex Education could be called Human Sexuality. A discussion of alcohol, tobacco, and drugs could be titled Mood Modifiers, or a mental health unit Psychic Ecology. The title of a unit should arouse the student's curiosity and create interest. A creative and dynamic curriculum begins with exciting topics.

Are there other topics not included in the traditional health curriculum which could make the course more relevant and prepare students to face future experiences that will affect their mental and physical well-being? Could we introduce a unit, for instance, on death education and suicide prevention? Why not include a unit on psychic phenomena, or one called Health in the Year 2000?

Try Micro-Courses

On the other hand, the present curriculum, based on a unit concept, may not be the proper way to teach health. A school using this concept may require a one-unit health education course for graduation. In such a school, ninth-grade students might attend health education classes five days a week for one semester. I would like to propose a student-centered rather than a teacher-centered approach to curriculum offerings. Under this approach, a variety of micro-courses would be offered in the curriculum. Students could meet the one-semester requirement by selecting any three 6-week micro-courses any time between their freshman and senior years. This approach is based on the belief that we in health education cannot accomplish all of the objectives for our courses in the limited time allotted to us. What we end up with is 100% cognitive learning, with no success in the affective domain or action domain. I agree with Toffler when he states that "children should be permitted far greater choice than at present [in selecting their curriculum]; they should be encouraged to taste a wide variety of short-term courses."[2] Such experiences should be based on present as well as future needs.

Certain courses based totally on behavioral change can be offered in school curriculums. I can conceive of short-term courses on weight control, smoking, abuse, or physical fitness, and action programs pertaining to ecology. Some of these experiences, if used as micro-courses, could be offered in the evening when students could take them with their parents. I can foresee parent-child courses in weight control, nutrition, or physical fitness. It seems that there would be a wealth of potential in this type of curriculum offering.

Get Involved in the Community

Another suggestion is for a practicum course in which students would be actively engaged in a community project pertaining to the improvement of the health of their community. Students should also be given the opportunity to receive health education credit by working in a local hospital as a candy striper, working with patients as a volunteer in a medical care facility, helping with cancer crusades, etc. These learning experiences under the supervision of qualified people, coordinated by the school health educator, could be extremely relevant and educational for the student. Another good idea would be to include a course on ecology, or maybe a reading class in health education. In addition, I would like to suggest that an advanced course at the junior or senior level be offered to students on an elective basis to explore in depth a variety of health-related topics. This could be offered during the summer when the instructor could take the class on weekend camping trips and in an outdoor situation informally introduce and discuss ideas pertinent to the health of both themselves and society.

Let Students Do the Teaching

Students can teach a health education course. Students learn in a variety of ways—from teachers, from materials, from experiences, and from other students. Much of what a student learns comes from his peer group; some of the most meaningful learning is from personal experience. It is unfortunate that many curriculums do not offer opportunities for these types of learning experiences. In a course centered around students teaching students, the teacher could identify five or six students who have leadership abilities and work with them individually to lead small groups of their peers. This gives students responsibility and personalizes the instruction. This approach could be especially useful in large classes.

There are a number of opportunities for creativity in health education curriculum design. The ideas presented in this article are intended to stimulate some thinking on the part of the reader. We have only scratched the surface in looking for innovations in health education curriculum development.

[1] Alvin Toffler. *Future Shock.* New York: Bantam Books, 1970. p. 409.
[2] *Ibid.*, p. 412.

Vary Your Teaching Methods

GLEN G. GILBERT is an assistant professor of health education, P.O. Box 751, Portland State University, Portland, Oregon 97207.

Teachers of health education consistently ask two basic questions about the desirability of using innovative teaching methods. These questions have been raised during numerous inservice workshops over the last few years: (1) why should we provide a variety of teaching methods? and (2) how can we provide such a variety of teaching methods? The answers to both questions are extremely important and any competent health educator should be able to answer both questions.

An answer to the first question can be proposed after referring to what the experts in the field have to say about the need for variety in teaching methods. These authorities draw conclusions based on research and personal experience. They agree that providing a variety of teaching methods is important if we are to enhance the learning setting and to overcome any stigma attached to health education as the result of historical sins committed during the presentation of health education information. In addition, the following are important reasons for providing a variety of teaching methods.

1. An interesting methodology prevents many discipline problems. Students who are interested in what they are doing are much less likely to act inappropriately in the classroom. This holds true for adult students as well as younger students.

2. It is a teacher's responsibility to provide an educational environment. This means teachers must do whatever is necessary and within their capabilities to motivate students to favorably alter health behavior; experience indicates that it is not an easy task. If teachers must stand on their heads to reach the students, then they should do it. Certainly we cannot reach every student, but we can reach many. We cannot all be showmen or great orators, but we should do all we can to favorably alter health behavior.

3. The performance of students is one reflection of teaching performance. If students are not performing well then much of the responsibility must be assumed by the teacher involved. Certainly it is a joint responsibility (student and teacher), but a large part of it must lie with the nature of the instruction. Utilizing appropriate methods is likely to increase student performance.

4. You can make anything *worth learning* interesting. If the material you are presenting is truly worth learning then you should be able to develop a strategy whereby the worth becomes evident to your students. Teachers must be willing to face the fact that they may be presenting irrelevant information. If you can't readily demonstrate that the information you are presenting is relevant, you had better take another look at that information and perhaps update or eliminate it.

How do we provide a variety of relevant teaching methods? Numerous texts have been written on the subject in health education, as well as in other fields. One technique found very helpful is to determine objectives to be achieved, then review the following chart of strategies and make a decision as to which might best facilitate the achievement of stated objectives.

This chart was developed by me for use with pre-service and in-service teachers. Each method is rated as to the likelihood of that particular method accomplishing various types of objectives. The ratings listed in three columns to the right of the method are: "MF" meaning most frequently; "O" meaning occasionally; or if blank, it is highly unlikely that it would be used in such a manner.

Objectives written in the cognitive domain generally require recall of information (e.g., the student will be able to list the seven danger signs of cancer). Affective objectives generally require an analysis of feelings or perhaps result in an attitude modification (e.g., the student will indicate her willingness to assume her part of the responsibility for early detection of cancer by reporting any unusual findings to her doctor immediately without waiting for regular checkups or pain). Psychomotor objectives require action (not just writing and thinking) during the activity or result in the student carrying out a physical action (e.g., the student will be able to demonstrate on Resusci-Anne correct mouth-to-mouth resuscitation). Additional information on objectives is readily available in any of the methods books listed in the bibliography.

It is suggested that the reader or student keep clearly in mind the objectives to be achieved by a class or course, then review the list, checking those methods which might achieve stated objectives. Following such an appraisal, consider how each checked method might be implemented and then make a decision based on feasibility and likelihood of successful accomplishment of objectives. Following these guidelines should discourage selection based only on ease of use and will encourage innovation.

Using this system an appropriate technique should be located if the material being covered is useful and important. The reader may notice an overabundance of available cognitive teaching methods. It generally requires more preparation and thought on the part of the teacher in order to utilize techniques which influence attitudes and stimulate action.

This article has presented a rationale for employing a variety of teaching methods and has presented a list of methods to achieve that end. If readers are unfamiliar with any of the teaching methods, they may wish to review some of the sources in the bibliography and/or correspond with the author.

Summary of teaching methods and strategies according to likelihood of meeting objectives in cognitive, affective and psychomotor domains

	Cognitive Knowledge	Affective Attitude	Psychomotor Action
1. Music	MF	O	O
2. Cartoons	MF	MF	
3. Brainstorming & buzz sessions	MF	O	O
4. Stories with fill-in-the blanks	MF	O	
5. Interviews	MF	O	
6. Pantomimes	MF	O	MF
7. Self-appraisal	O	MF	O
8. Panel discussions	MF	O	
9. Visits to agencies	O	O	
10. Field trips	O	O	
11. Bulletin boards, displays, flannel boards	MF	O	
12. Transparencies	MF	O	
13. Review bees	MF		
14. Value clarification	O	MF	O
15. Mystery puzzles	MF		
16. Word-o-games	MF		
17. Anagrams	MF		
18. Crossword puzzles	MF		
19. Games	MF	O	O
20. Simulated situations or critical incidents	MF	MF	MF
21. Problem solutions (a specific technique)		MF	
22. Mock radio and T.V.	MF	MF	O
23. Personal health improvement projects	O	MF	MF
24. Student produced movies, slides, or videotapes	MF	O	O
25. Debates	MF	O	O
26. Skits	MF	O	
27. Plays	MF	O	
28. Role playing	O	MF	
29. Self-tests	MF		
30. Surveys	O	MF	
31. Oral reports (individual or group)	MF	O	O
32. Guest speakers	MF	MF	
33. Computer assisted instruction	MF		
34. Programmed learning	MF		
35. Experiments	MF	O	MF
36. Demonstrations	MF	O	MF
37. Mobiles	MF		
38. Charts, transparencies or graphs	MF		
39. Models	MF		
40. Slides	MF	MF	O
41. Videotapes	MF	O	O
42. Auditory tapes or records	MF	O	O
43. Films and film strips	MF	O	O

MF= Most frequently
O= Occasionally
   If blank, it is rarely or never used in this way.

Bibliography

Bedworth, David A. and Bedworth, Albert E. *Health Education: A Process for Human Effectiveness.* New York: Harper and Row, 1978.

Burt, John and Meeks, Linda. *Education for Sexuality.* 2nd ed. Philadelphia: W. B. Saunders, 1974.

Engs, Ruth, et al. *Health Games Students Play: Creative Strategies for Health Education,* Dubuque, IA: Kendall/Hunt, 1975.

Ensor, Phyllis. *Instructor's Resource and Methods Handbook for Health Education,* Rockleigh, NJ: Allyn and Bacon, 1975.

Fodor, John and Dalis, Gus. *Health Instruction: Theory and Application,* Philadelphia: Lea and Febiger, 1974.

Green, Lawrence. ''Determining the Impact and Effectiveness of Health Education as it Relates to Federal Policy,'' prepared for the office of the Deputy Assistant Secretary for Planning and Evaluation/Health, H.E.W., rev. April 1976.

Hoover, Kenneth, *The Professional Teachers Handbook,* Rockleigh, NJ: Allyn and Bacon, 1975.

Kime, Robert; Schlaadt, Richard; and Tritsch, Leonard. *Health Instruction: An Action Approach,* Englewood Cliffs, NJ: Prentice-Hall, 1977.

Lemeke, John. *278 Experimental Strategies for Instructors of Health,* Dubuque, IA: Kendall/Hunt, 1975.

Oberteuffer, Delbert, *School Health Education,* New York: Harper and Row, 1972.

Read, Donald and Greene, Walter, *Creative Teaching in Health,* New York, Macmillan, 1975.

Russell, Robert, *Health Education,* Washington, DC: AAHPER, 1975.

Sorochan, Walter, *Personal Health Appraisal,* New York: John Wiley and Sons, 1976.

Willgoose, Carl, *Health Teaching in Secondary Schools,* Philadelphia: W. B. Saunders, 1972.

Films for Effective Affective Teaching

JAMES R. MULLEN is a teacher of English at the Lower Cape May County Regional High School, Cape May, New Jersey 08204.

One of the most significant educational trends of the last decade is the movement toward what is generally known as affective or humanistic education. With roots in the humanistic psychology of Abraham Maslow and human-potential growth centers like the Esalen Institute, humanistic and affective education (the terms are virtually interchangeable) deals with the growth of the whole person—the development of sensory awareness, interpersonal relations, and, perhaps most important, self-awareness and self-knowledge. Every board of education in every city and town in the country has some general statement of goals for the development of the whole person (usually couched in terms of encouraging "good citizenship" and "sound mind"). But in most schools, these goals are empty pieties. Often the best a teacher can do is to try to bring students up to grade, to advance students in basic skills, and maintain a semblance of order. Issues such as drug abuse, lack of interest, disruptive behavior, and poor retention are increasing.

The time has come, more and more educational reformers believe, for affective education to assume its rightful place alongside the more traditional curriculum. One of the main obstacles to this kind of change, however, is a dearth of good, proven materials. Teachers in search of a geography book to use in their classes can choose from hundreds, and huge film catalogs are readily available. But if a teacher tries to find a text or film on affective education, he'd better have some inside information.

One illustration of how useful materials on affective education can be when they are available is a program developed by a small firm of psychologists and film makers in New York City. The company, Film Modules Inc., is being funded by the National Institute of Mental Health, the New York State Department of Education, and the New

York State Narcotic Addiction Control Commission under the umbrella title "Drug Abuse Self-Awareness." Four separate programs for school-related use have been made available.

Each program in the self-awareness series is based on a concept of film usage which was developed by producer-therapist Robert Rubin. The concept's first application was a stress training program for police officers. It has been interposed within the training programs of more than 150 police departments throughout the country since its release in 1970.

The basic premise of Rubin's work is that in most cases films do not elicit genuine involvement and feedback, but rather make of the viewer a passive observer who experiences the film vicariously, at best. Starting several years ago, Rubin began to explore ways of mak-

ing film a more directly involving medium. The "film modules," as he calls his films, are structured to demand specific kinds of feedback and interaction. The result is a remarkably efficient, yet gentle generator of mature behavior.

The heart of each program is a series of film modules that focus on situations of tremendous emotional intensity and which suddenly and unexpectedly stop, leaving the viewer so emotionally keyed up that he or she is likely to have an almost physical need for a discussion or a general exchange of feelings and reactions with others. As any teacher who has ever tried to experiment with group dynamics knows, simply saying to students, "Well, what do you feel—tell us about your feelings" is likely to elicit dead silence more than any other response. The film modules, on the other hand, make a verbal response a kind of necessary relief.

One indication of the success of this concept in forcing a genuine and often profound emotional feedback from students was the response to one of the drug abuse self-awareness films for high school students. A 17-minute module entitled "Fear" was tested with a group of high school teenagers selected at random in a rural school. The students were so eager to talk about their own experiences of fear in a variety of situations that the discussion became a kind of confessional. "I felt like I was experiencing it myself," said one boy referring to the module. "My heart was beating harder and I didn't know what to do. And I was breaking out in a sweat right while I was watching it. I had this feeling that everyone was trying to escape and I was left there by myself." "But," added another, "if you show your fear all the time as you feel it inside of you, then you're usually going to get caught. As you go along and you learn to deal with your fear, then it prepares you better for the next time. But if you let your fear run rampant, you go insane." A video tape was made of this discussion and it was obvious from a single viewing that the discussion included not only the recognition that the fear existed, but the more mature awareness that fear need not be a mastering emotion, that being "in touch" with one's emotions helps one to deal in a more realistic and adult way than if one were less aware.

As the title of the series implies, drug abuse is one target of the films. It is only an indirect target, however. Although each of the film modules in this series deals with teenagers using drugs in a peer-group situation, the emphasis is more on the common emotions and experiences of adolescent growth than on the usual sermonizing lecture so typical of drug prevention programs everywhere. If you really know who you are, the program says, if you're in touch with yourself and behaving in a mature and sensible way, drugs won't trouble you. It's only when your head gets messed up (as happens at times to the teenagers in the films) that drugs might cause you trouble. The real key to the drug problem, in short, is not lecturing and punishment, but human self-understanding and self-concept.

A great deal of the success of Rubin's film modules and the supportive material must be credited to his talents as a filmmaker. The films have a quality of such complete honesty and spontaneity that it's difficult to believe they were made from written scripts and performed by teenage actors in New Jersey and Long Island—that they aren't real-life documentaries. The scripts and dialogue are based on hundreds of hours of taped group probes with teachers and young people, often the same kids who later performed in the films. It is easy, therefore, for most teenagers in settings varying from urban to semi-rural to identify strongly with the experiences and feelings presented.

Rubin sees his films as merely one component in a total educational program, and there are extensive teacher guides, intended to be used in a package of twelve lessons but adaptable to a number of different formats. The supportive written materials which guide the leader in the use of the films are so explicit that a teacher (or peer leader) who has never had any experience with group dynamics or affective curriculum can follow them easily. In line with the more process-oriented goals of affective education (as contrasted with the product-oriented goals of traditional education), the introduction to the teacher's guide states: "The main task for the leader . . . when using the film modules is to unlearn, or at least temporarily suspend, what you know about teaching. There is no *knowledge* which you can *teach* in this program." The instructions proceed with such suggestions as (in connection with "Fear") "Ask for volunteers to share personal stories with the others about when they were 'conned' into doing something they were afraid to do and did it anyway." Or (in connection with "Humiliation and Anger") "Keep the discussion on target: 'How would it feel if you were turned in?' 'Did anything like that ever happen to you?'." The teacher's guide includes a series of student work sheets which help students apply what they learn about themselves to real life behavior.

Although the film modules are definitely not product-oriented, they do have specific educational objectives. The teacher's guide explicitly states, for example, that it is desirable to establish that "mature behavior involves making a clear distinction between a feeling and an action." The guide also stresses the importance of peer-group pressure in shaping discussions to examine feelings objectively and the necessity of creating an open, honest, and relaxed classroom atmosphere (with helpful suggestions on how to do this). In various experimental sessions with the films, students quickly realized many of these objectives by themselves. "As you go along and learn to deal with your fear," one boy in a high school in Schenectady said during a discussion of "Fear," "it prepares you better for the next time."

The films also open the way for some benefits not mentioned in the specific lesson plans. When one teacher in a high school on Long Island used the films, the most striking result he noted was that for the first time the students who favored drugs and those who opposed them were talking to each other and communicating. "Before, no matter what I did, they didn't want to communicate with each other," the teacher said. "Many of the drug users said they needed drugs to communicate, but it emerged during the discussion that they were communicating effectively in the discussion without drugs. That really surprised them."

As for other specific results, the teacher couldn't be sure—"It's still in their minds," he commented several weeks after showing the films. "I don't expect it to provoke permanent change, but they keep referring to the films in all kinds of contexts. It seems to have definitely planted seeds. I've used a great deal of audiovisual material, and this is by far the most effective."

"We spent a lot of time talking about feelings and emotions," commented another teacher who has also used the films. "For a large number of them it really hit home. Lots of kids get completely turned off when adults start discussing drugs—for the last four or five years that's all they've heard. There was none of that when we used the film modules; they could identify with the kids completely."

Another unexpected benefit emerged in a mainly black and Puerto Rican school district in New York City. There are few minority-group teenagers in the films—they were intended mainly for a middle-class suburban audience, and the leader of this particular inner-city drug program reports that students who had seen the films in her district were delighted to observe that for a change the poor and the minorities are not depicted as being closely associated with "the drug problem." Seeing drug abuse not as a racial issue helped to calm the defensiveness and hostility displayed toward most drug programs.

In addition to the high school series, the company has also produced a series on drug abuse self-awareness for teachers, another program for parents, and a single film for students in elementary school that clears up many common misconceptions and unreal fears.

Affective Teaching

Many educators quite legitimately question the role of schools in psychological education. Affective gains are difficult, if not impossible, to measure. Therefore, are such materials safe when used by the average teacher? "Maybe affective education isn't much different from a bull session—and shouldn't school be more than bull sessions?"

The film modules programs offer only a brief immersion in intensive techniques for developing self-awareness, and their positive effects, if left unsupported, will dissipate with time. A learning system has been devised as a follow-up, called "role modules." Here the students reenact (using role playing techniques) the situations presented in the role modules. The goal is twofold, first to reinforce the emotional awarenesses they had attained earlier from the films, and second, to present the many options available for mature behavior in real life.

One could argue that the teacher who would readily agree to use the film modules is probably someone already inclined to favor affective

education and to encourage a relaxed classroom atmosphere.

Whatever their emotional benefit, the programs are proving to be useful to a growing number of teachers. As one teacher put it, "They served as a perfect trigger for discussion; they helped to create a nonthreatening environment in which the kids felt free to talk about things that they were really concerned about." Rubin's film modules offer a workable alternative to Clifton Fadiman's illustrated lectures of Dickens. As any teacher who has watched his or her classes drift off in a cloud of boredom knows too well, it's the kind of alternative the schools desperately need.

THE END

Effective Teaching: Variety in the Classroom

MARY SUTHERLAND is a master of public health student at the University of Tennessee, Knoxville, Tennessee 37916.
WILLIAM HEMMER is an associate professor in the Department of Health Science, State University College-Brockport, Brockport, New York 14420.

In developing an evaluation procedure for assessing student teacher competencies in a competency based teacher education program, checklists of what the student teacher is expected to do using a variety of techniques have been developed by a consortium of teachers, administrators, and college supervisors of the State University College at Brockport school health program. The field testing of this instrument was conducted with approximately 30 supervising teachers and student teachers. The participants provided many suggestions for the improvement of the assessment instrument, adding components and subtracting others.

All the clues to the qualities of a good lesson are provided for the student teacher before the lesson is planned. Since the clues can be built into the lesson plan the lesson will be better than if student teachers are left to their own devices to develop a good lesson. Therefore, the Competency Evaluation Packet helps the student teacher prepare sound, well-planned lessons which will succeed in the classroom.

Supervising teachers found that they were able to benefit by the checklists of expectations developed and found that their teaching improved because they were conscious of the essential ingredients of a particular type of lesson. A checklist of the qualities which the group felt would ensure success for three types of lessons follows with a discussion of the checklist items.

Demonstration Lesson

The teachers should demonstrate successfully, all of the following.
1. Arouse students' interest and attention before starting.
2. Explain the purpose of the demonstration.
3. Demonstrate the steps in logical order.
4. Explain the purpose of the various steps.
5. Provide clarifying material to the students.
6. Hold the attention of the students.
7. Provide sufficient opportunity for student questions.
8. Give clear answers to student questions.
9. Evaluate the success of the demonstration by eliciting student feedback.

As in any lesson, the teacher must begin by catching the imagination of the students so they will begin to pay attention. Students should know why this idea is being demonstrated. Logical order is important so that students can follow the procedure and understand the reason for each step, as well as, what is happening at each state in the demonstration. Thus, an explanation of the purpose of the steps as the demonstration proceeds is helpful as are any clarifying materials. Clarifying materials can be anything from references to things in the students' own textbook to definitions written on the chalkboard.

The teacher should keep things moving along so students' attention does not wander. This requires enthusiasm, showmanship, and ham acting. Another thing that breaks the monotony of the teacher's voice and helps to hold interest is encouraging student questions as the demonstration moves along. There is nothing like clear, concise answers to encourage more questions which means the teacher must be well prepared to field the types of questions which may arise. At the end of the demonstration, the teacher will want to elicit student feedback, probably with a few questions, such as: What do you think has happened here? Why? Do you agree with this explanation? Why do you suppose we did (this) instead of (that)? What might have happened if we had done (this) at (step 1)? Why?

The teacher evaluates the success of the lesson by probing the depths of the students' understanding of what has happened in the demonstration they have just seen.

Dramatization Lesson

Teachers should be able to demonstrate successfully, all of the following.

1. Arouse students' interests and attention before starting.
2. Select a relevant situation for student participation involving one main idea or issue. This could involve personalities related to an individual's beliefs, hopes, and aspirations.
3. Select students who are well informed on the issues and are self-confident in performing before their peers.
4. Prepare the class in what to look for in the dramatization, e.g. behaviors, feelings, etc.
5. Actively involve the students in the dramatization, but maintain orderly direction toward fulfillment of the objectives.
6. Evaluate the dramatization as it relates to the objectives by means of review, discussions or question-answer sessions.

Again the teacher must have a device for getting students' attention before starting. If the situation to be dramatized is familiar and important to the students, if somehow the students can relate to one or more of the characters, interest can be sustained. Usually situations or ideas which relate to their values, beliefs, or hopes are considered relevant topics by students.

In selecting the actors and actresses for a dramatization, whether it be impromptu or prepared ahead of time, it is important to use volunteers who are self-confident in front of their peers. Nothing kills a dramatization like a shy student who mumbles a few words and quickly tries to sit down because he would rather be almost anywhere except in front of the classroom. The participants in the demonstration should also be those who are well informed on the issues presented and who can easily visualize the situation to be dramatized. This is especially true in impromptu role playing.

Students in their seats should be given a charge by the teacher to look for certain behaviors, feelings, or whatever. The audience should be given an important evaluative or observer role so they will not feel like passive observers, but co-participants in a class enterprise.

Objectives should be made clear to students so they will know why they are doing this dramatization. At the end of the lesson, the teacher should evaluate the dramatization in light of the objectives. Again, a five or ten minute discussion of what happened may be crucial in getting the main point of the lesson across to students. The teacher, for example, might ask: Was the dramatization realistic? Why or why not? Do you think (the protagonist) acted realistically? Why? Would you have said (or acted) as (a character) did? Why? If not, how would you have acted in this situation? How could the dramatization have been improved? Did you ever see anything like this happen in real life? Where? How?

Audiovisual Lesson

Teachers should be able to do all of the following.

1. Explain the purpose of using the audiovisual material to the students.
2. Pose questions for students to seek answers to during the presentation.
3. Use questions to get students to think about material during or after the presentation.
4. Select audiovisual material which will increase the students' depth of understanding and learning of the curriculum content.
5. Involve students in the interpretation of the message presented in the media.
6. Relate the media's message to the curriculum objective.
7. Select media which present the message in an effective manner.
8. Select media with appropriate vocabulary level for the students.
9. Help the children conceptualize.
10. Summarize the main instructional purposes of the media.

Whether filmstrip, 16mm film, film loop, slides or large poster pictures, the teacher should first explain to the students why they are being asked to look listen to it. In other words, the lesson objectives should be made clear. To involve students and support the purpose explained, ask students several questions in advance, keyed into the objective. One or two questions given in advance are generally all that students can keep in mind. An alternative is for the teacher to pose the questions one at a time during the presentation of the audiovisual material.

The important thing is to get the students to think critically or to inquire about the material being presented, both during the presentation process and afterward. Of course, for worthwhile thinking to be stimulated, the audiovisual material must be carefully selected to focus the students' attention on the objective desired and to foster learning of the content of the curriculum.

The questions and the teaching procedures used should be designed to involve the students in interpreting the media's message. This involvement should encourage creative solutions to problems and interpretation of phenomena and events depicted. The opportunity to use creative abilities sparks the interest and enthusiasm of the students in the project at hand. If possible, the teacher must skillfully allow the media's message to be related to the curriculum objective by the student instead of by the teacher.

The media which present the message effectively are usually best for stimulating student interest through the use of open ended questions. A straight factual presentation makes student involvement difficult since the media seems to be saying, "Here it is folks, this is the way it is, there's no argument possible with these facts." Students, not being subject matter experts, are usually in awe of straight factual presentations and are not able to challenge this type of presentation effectively.

If the media has audio or printed components, the teacher must make sure the vocabulary level is appropriate for the students—not too simple or too hard.

The teacher will want to help the children conceptualize the main objective of the lesson, usually by followup questions that help students understand and evaluate what they have just seen. These followup questions will also help to summarize the main instructional purpose of the media presentation.

Conclusion

Teachers who want to do demonstration, dramatizations, or audiovisual lessons for added variety in their classrooms will find these checklists an aid in remembering all the fine points that are essential for making a lesson click with a class of students. The checklists can be applied profitably both before and after the lesson. Before the lesson, they can be used as a guide in planning so that all necessary components are built into the lesson. After the lesson a teacher can use this same checklist as a thoughtful means of evaluating his/her performance in the classroom. In the light of this evaluation technique, apparent weaknesses can be shored up by extra effort in the planning stage the next time a particular type of lesson is attempted.

Health Science Fairs

HENRY A. LASCH is professor of health science, Department of Physical Education, New Mexico State University, Las Cruces, New Mexico 88003.

Science fairs have been a traditional project in many school districts throughout the United States, reaching a peak of interest after the space-age touched off a fervor of activity in the mathematics and science curricula.

We are now on the threshold of a new era in the health sciences. The crises brought on by drug abuse, the venereal disease epidemic, smoking, alcoholism, destruction of the environment, and other problems have increased public awareness in health. Although it is deplorable that most schools and communities waited for crises to develop before they realized the importance of a comprehensive health program, we are on the brink of one of the greatest expansions in health in the history of public education. Every possible means must be employed to convey the message of school health to the public.

The health science fair is one type of activity that will add new dimensions to school health education. It is similar to the traditional science fair except that it is limited to projects and exhibits which portray health as the central theme. Schools that may not want to sponsor separate health science fairs could designate health as the main topic in their regular science fair. Whatever route is taken, the end results should be worthwhile.

In organizing health science fairs it should be recognized that any type of project can be included as long as it pertains to health. It may cover anything ranging from personal and community health affairs to world-wide health problems. Special emphasis should be given to projects related to health and medical research and current, scientific developments affecting man's health and longevity.

Why Sponsor a Health Fair?

The health science fair presents an unrivaled opportunity to promote greater health awareness among students, school personnel, and the community as a whole. Greater understanding of the importance and scope of health in a changing world can be gained from this type of enterprise. Students may discover new interests and meaning in health and unlimited opportunities exist for creativity in all areas of health. Students who exhibit genuine interest and enthusiasm may show promise for careers in one of the many allied health and medical professions. It is quite conceivable that some of the critical health manpower shortage could be reduced if students were provided opportunities to develop their interests and creative talents in the field of health at an earlier age.

As plans take shape for a health science fair, students should become aware of the multitude of topics and programs which comprise school health, public health, and international health. A health science fair permits greater student involvement in current health affairs. It can also serve as a valuable tool to publicize health among all segments of the community. Education must search for better ways to challenge and stimulate the minds of youth in the diversified fields of health.

The health science fair is an effective way to gain respect for the entire discipline as well as a means of securing more public support for health as a separate subject in the secondary schools. Certain projects can focus on health hazards and deficiencies in the community, thus providing students with a challenge to assist in the solution of current health problems.

Guidelines for Projects

1. All projects entered in the fair should center around some area of health. The theme of the project should be clearly defined and described.

2. Students should select their own projects as long as basic rules and guidelines are followed. These should be clearly established by students and faculty.

3. Projects should be designed by the students, who should be expected to do their own construction and assembling.

4. The general plan of the projects should be approved by a committee of students and teachers.

5. Both individual and group projects should be encouraged.

6. Participants in the fair should be limited to one project in order to strengthen the quality of entries.

Organizational Committees

A health science fair will have a greater possibility of success if committee responsibility is clearly defined and overlapping is avoided. The general administration of the fair can be handled by a steering committee. Other suggested committees are: publicity, design and construction, finance, facilities, and judging. Additional committees may be added as deemed necessary.

Final success of a health science fair will depend upon the cooperation of all committees, the enthusiasm of those who participate in the planning, the motivation of student and public interest, time allowed for adequate preparation of projects, selection of a desirable site, and the continuous publicity given the entire project.

THE OPEN CONTRACT—
A PROGRAM OF
INDIVIDUALIZED STUDY

B. E. PRUITT is a staff member at Lewisville High School, Lewisville, Texas 75067

As a multidisciplinary topic, health education can offer an excellent opportunity to make classroom experiences germaine to individual life styles. Unlike many other areas of study, health education is not obligated to concentrate on fragmented tools which may, or may not, be used to affect life quality. Instead, classroom health offers a chance to experience concepts of living—the "big ideas" of responsible personal health.

At Lewisville High School, we have recognized this opportunity and are attempting to offer classroom health to our students to not only provide them with information about healthful living but to do this in a learning environment which emphasizes individual application of health related information. We have developed a program of individual study, the "open contract." The goal of the open contract program is to provide an environment in which each participant successfully identifies topics or problems within specific health-related areas, acquires information about them, and, by analyzing the gathered information, proposes possible means of dealing with such topics or problems. The ambiguity of this goal is necessary if the vast range of individual differences and needs is to be considered.

Participants in the open contract program are employed as student investigators for 18 weeks. During that time they are considered free citizens within the program. They assume three primary responsibilities: selection of topics or problems for study, selection of methods of investigation or investigation categories, and selection of grades.

Selection of Topics

Participants in the open contract program are free to select topics for investigation, but they are restricted in two ways. They must choose topics within the areas of study established at the beginning of the program, generally corresponding to the basic areas recommended in the Texas Education Agency's Bulletin 691, *Secondary School Health Education Curriculum Guide.* The second restriction is that each selection must be appropriately limited to be effectively dealt with through investigation procedures established by the investigation categories. A topic such as "food" is obviously too broad to be effectively investigated, but a topic such as "food fads" is more appropriate. The teacher never decides what topics are to be studied, for in doing so he would risk losing the individual emphasis of the program. Rather, he establishes boundaries within which the student is encouraged to select any topic or problem of personal interest.

Selection of Investigation Categories

Once a student has chosen a topic for study he must then select a method of investigation from the investigation categories established by the teacher at the beginning of the program. They must vary in degree of difficulty and value so the student has several choices. A more difficult category may be valued as much as 10 points while a simple category is worth only 5 points. When selecting an investigation category the student must consider how much work he wishes to do with the topic, how many points he wishes to earn, and whether the topic and the method of investigation are compatible.

Following are several examples of possible investigation categories, designed for the ninth grade level and currently a part of the program for Health I students at Lewisville High School. (With a more advanced student, more involved investigation procedures would be appropriate.) The six examples will be explained in relation to the open contract design.

Position Paper: Each six-week period includes three opportunities for the student investigator to express opinions on controversial topics. This expression is done in the form of a position paper. Such statements of personal opinion allow a student to receive credit for investigating his own thinking in the areas of study. The position papers are graded according to how well the selected topic relates to the area of study, the topic is covered, the arguments are presented, and its general tidiness. The maximum value for any position paper is five points.

Critique: The critique category is provided so the student investigator can receive credit for analyzing the variety of information found in the health field. Newspaper and magazine articles, books, films, television programs, or personal interviews all provide opportunities for developing critiques. The student is encouraged to produce a piece of creative evaluation of both the information and the information source. Each critique is valued at eight points and is graded according to how the information relates to the area of study, how a summary of the information is presented, how an analysis of the information is carried out, how the source is identified (usually through a bibliographic note) and its neatness.

Correspondence: In each six-week period, students have three opportunities to receive credit for corresponding with various public health agencies or businesses concerning health-related information. This optional investigation category exposes the student to the variety of agencies, businesses, and associations which are concerned with the health of their clientele and helps the student encounter samples of literature provided by such service organizations. Students are provided with a list of appropriate agencies with which they may correspond. Each correspondence is valued at five points, credited when evidence of the correspondence is presented. As long as the information requested relates to the areas of study, full credit is given.

Examination: Three optional examinations worth up to eight points each are provided every six weeks. Questions are usually essay and deal with class activities, suggested readings, or general information to which the student may have been exposed. What might seem to be a misnomer in referring to examinations as one of the investigation categories is not so when examinations are looked upon as individual investigations of personal knowledge. Students are encouraged to write examinations with this in mind.

Individual Project: The category "individual project" gives the student investigator a chance to express his creativity, expand his knowledge in a health-related topic, and receive credit at the same time.

The design and means of development of the project are entirely up to the student. Bulletin boards, book reports, or special notebooks are common projects. Originality, however, is encouraged. Up to ten points credit may be earned each six-week period by the completion of this investigation category.

Committee Project: If three or more student investigators wish to work together on a project, they may choose to complete the category "committee project." The only restrictions are that only one project may be completed during any one six-week period and the selected topic must relate to the area of study. Each member of a committee may receive a maximum of ten points for a project.

Most, but not all, points are earned through investigation procedures. Up to 30 points may be earned each six-week period through class participation. Regular activities are planned which involve group work, role playing, or guest speakers so that information is provided over areas of study. Many activities are designed to help students with their investigations, or for the sole purpose of having fun with health. The credit available encourages students to take advantage of the activities or to make use of the class time provided for investigating chosen topics.

A progress record is used to maintain a running account of the number of points earned by each participant in the open contract program. An official and an unofficial progress record is kept for each of the three six-week periods during the program. The unofficial record is kept up to date by each student investigator so that he is always aware of where he stands. The official record is placed in a file and kept up to date by the teacher. Official credit is recorded at the time individual investigations are placed on file. At the end of each six-week period, the total of all points recorded on the official record is determined, and the resulting number is the six-week grade.

Selection of Grades

If a student investigator chooses to complete an investigation option, he does not automatically receive full credit. But, points are never subtracted from a student's grade. This evident contradiction leads us to one of the most important aspects of the open contract program—the grading technique.

A major criticism of the traditional classroom environment involves the extremely negative approach used in grading. When averaging is used, one poor grade may destroy all incentive. The open

contract program, on the other hand, involves a completely positive approach. When an investigation is graded it is awarded points for things done well; no points are subtracted for mistakes. For example, if a student completes the investigation category "critique I," he may receive up to 8 points. When grading the presentation the teacher notes any areas in which the critique may be improved. If the teacher feels that the paper is well done then a full 8 points may be awarded. If the teacher sees ways for improvement he may award 4 points or 2 points, depending on the amount of improvement necessary. Any time less than the maximum number of points are awarded, the

student has the option of accepting the points awarded by placing the paper on file, or of rejecting the points, making the indicated improvements, and resubmitting the paper to be graded again. If a student is not satisfied with this grade the paper may be reworked once again.

Usually when students rework a category, they improve the number of points earned. If, however, a second presentation receives a lower grade than the first, the student may ask that the first be filed and the original points awarded. Once points are recorded they must not be subtracted. The student is encouraged in every way to earn the highest grade possible.

Final grades are determined by the total number of points accumulated during the 18 week session. A student receives a good grade after completing a certain number of investigation categories well. A poor grade is given when the student chooses to complete fewer investigation categories. The option is available to complete no investigations and fail. This too is considered a respectable choice because the student is held responsible for his decisions.

This totally positive grading technique is essential to the success of the open contract program. The student must feel responsible for his own grade and he can feel that way only if he is allowed the option of correcting and improving his work in each category to a point of personal satisfaction.

Most participants in the open contract program have responded positively to this individualized motivational approach. They have become deeply involved in a variety of health-related areas and, in general, have increased understanding of numerous concepts of healthful living. Perhaps more importantly, however, participants have enjoyed their health education experience.

THE MANY FACES OF ROLE PLAYING

LYNN TEPER-SINGER is an assistant professor in the Departments of Health Science, Physical Education, and Guidance and Counseling at Long Island University—The Brooklyn Center, Brooklyn, New York 11201.

Role playing as a classroom technique has provided a marvelous environment for the exploration of health concepts. In the February 1971 issue of *School Health Review* a step by step procedure of the traditional role playing situation was presented in an article entitled, "Role Playing as a Tool in Mental Health Education." Briefly the steps included:

1. *Sensitizing the group*—present a situation where the class discovers that each person perceives a given situation differently based on past experience, assumptions, and expectations

2. *The Warmup*—describe the role playing situation with limited information

3. *The Enactment*—spontaneous dramatization

4. *The Replay*—the same people switching roles

5. *Student Observation*—discussion by the students about their reactions

6. *The Evaluation*—draw conclusions

At this time I would like to present three alternative approaches to role playing. Although any area in mental health can be explored through these procedures, the following are examples for use in drug education.

Example I

Structure: The class is divided into groups of four. Each group sits in a small circle within a large circle that the groups form.

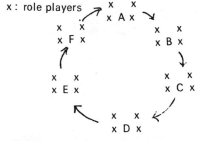

x : role players

Situation: Student arrives home to a family that has discovered a "stash" of drugs hidden away in his/her room.

Roles: Each group will enact the following roles spontaneously without preparation other than deciding on a role. Mother and/or father, brother and/or sister, student.

Procedure: In sequence each group performs their presentation of what they think will happen. (Group A then B then C, etc.) Generally each group has a different approach. The teacher may stop the group and go on to the next group at any point.

Discussion: After all groups have enacted their presentation, the teacher will have several options for proceeding with the discussion depending upon the material presented. Some possibilities include:

1. The class may form new groups based on the behavior displayed by the parents. Students who think their parents would behave as the role was played, would group together with the role players. For example: parent who cries "How could you do this to me"; parent who kicks child out; parent who questions with concern; parent who lectures and does not allow a response, etc.

Discussion questions may include: How do you feel when your parents approach you in this manner when they disapprove of your behavior? For what reasons do you believe your parents respond in this way? How would you approach your child if you were the parent?

2. The class may discuss their reaction to each group's performance.

3. The teacher may present questions for the small groups to discuss based on the diverse material that the teacher has been jotting down during the different presentations. For example:

Describe the ways in which the person caught responded.

For what reason do you believe people would respond in this way?

What information about drugs do you believe was false, which was factual?

What are the penalties for breaking drug laws?

What was your reaction when alcohol was mentioned as alright for the adults but "pot" was put down?

Example II

Structure: Single group performance with stop action directorship by the class. The performing group presents their interpretation of the situation in front of the class (the directors) who are sitting in a semi-circle around the classroom.

x- role players

o- directors

Situation: One student is trying to convince three friends to smoke a joint.

Roles: Person who does the convincing, person who refuses, person who is undecided, person who accepts.

Procedure: The group begins their enactment. At any point any member of the class, as well as the teacher, may stop the action by calling out "Stop Action" and

1. ask a question of a performer about how that performer feels at the moment.

2. assume the role of any of the players with a different approach.

3. ask the present players to switch roles.

Discussion: Questions for discussion may involve aspects dealing with group pressure and the decision-making process.

a. In what ways were the situations realistic or unrealistic?

b. How do you feel when someone tries to convince you to do something that you really don't wish to do?

c. What feelings do you have when you want to convince someone to do something and they refuse?

Example III

Structure: One individual sitting on the edge of the circle who will enact two opposing aspects of himself while the remaining members of the class listen.

x- role player
o- classmates

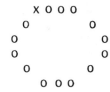

```
        x o o o
      o           o
    o               o
    o               o
      o           o
        o o o
```

Situation: The forces (feelings and attitudes) within the person that motivate him to use drugs versus those that influence him to refrain from using drugs.

Roles: The role is the dichotomy that exists within us that determines our decisions.

Procedure: The student holds up two hands (puppets may be used if appropriate for the age group). One hand is first used for emphasis "On the one hand why shouldn't I use drugs, everyone is doing it?" The other hand is then used "But on the other hand just because others do it doesn't mean I have to follow their example." The alternation of hands is repeated with each feeling and thought for or against the use of drugs.

Discussion: Questions for discussion may include:

1. In what ways are your feelings similar to and/or different from those presented?

2. What is your response in other situations where a conflict exists between your feelings, thoughts, and attitudes?

When teachers present role playing situations it is most important for them to have a facility for questioning so discussions are meaningful. The teacher's responsibility in role playing is essentially to help students identify and define what they are experiencing, as well as to help them investigate their feelings and reactions. A non-judgmental setting is therefore a must.

Suggestions for questioning:

1. Avoid questions that merely yield a yes or no response or that call for judgments such as good or bad, should or shouldn't.

2. Explore several ramifications of questions:

Clarify a point: If I understand you, you said. . . .

Seek additional information: Would you tell us more about this?

Evaluate: What do you think this might mean? How does the rest of the class feel about this?

Conclude: What happened? Why is this a problem? How could the outcome be altered?

3. Provide an atmosphere where questions arise from and between students as well as from you.

EXTRA CREDIT—
MAKE IT MEANINGFUL

GEORGE F. CARTER is an instructor in the Department of Health and Physical Education, Triton College, River Grove, Illinois 60171.

At one time or another most teachers from the elementary school through the university are confronted by students desiring to do an extra credit paper or project. Many times the student requesting the opportunity has fallen behind his classmates in regular assignments and would like to make amends through extra effort. In other words, the extra credit becomes a make-up which often causes problems for the instructor at or near the close of a term.

During the last nine years, many of my students at Triton College have requested extra credit in Science of Personal Health courses. Reasons for the request vary from the desire to achieve an A rather than a B, to pass rather than fail. Most requests have been made in the last week or two of the semester with little thought given to the learning experience. As a teacher, it is always encouraging to have a student request to do something extra but not under these circumstances. On the other hand, it is undesirable from an instructional viewpoint to deny a student a second opportunity, especially when they have requested the chance.

In the competition for grades, class rank, and as an opportunity to promote learning, the extra credit assignment should be used as a teaching strategy and should be open to all students. The nature of the assignment and appropriate grade compensation should be in keeping with the regular course evaluation procedures. Everything pertaining to extra credit should be carefully explained

to the students so that misunderstanding is held to a minimum.

So students understand how they are to be evaluated in health class, students are told the objective criteria used in evaluating their effort. Every effort is made to present the student with the opportunity to earn points toward his eventual grade. All assigned work is given a numerical value and students are made aware of the point value for tests, term projects, abstracts, oral reports, attendance, etc.

Extra credit is not used to replace regular work but to increase opportunities for willing students. The information given to each student enrolled in Science of Personal Health as a handout is shown here. Over the last several years this handout has been revised and it will be continually revised. There is no longer the urgent need for an extra credit project; the extra credit must be carefully planned and contribute to the learning experience of the student.

EXTRA CREDIT OPPORTUNITIES
Science of Personal Health
Dr. George F. Carter, Instructor

Students who are interested in improving their information and skill level are invited to submit extra credit projects. All projects must conform to the established guidelines for compensation. All points earned through extra effort will be added to the previously earned point total. Generally speaking, first come, first served on topics. All work must be in good form to be considered.

1. Students may report information gleaned from reading a newspaper or magazine article which covers the subject being discussed in class. The student must have a copy of the article to present to the instructor and give a brief account of the information to the class. Articles not pertaining to the day's lesson will not count as extra credit. (2 pts.)

2. Students may visit a local, county, or state health agency and make an oral report to the class about the visit. In addition, a one page summary of the visit, person visited, and other pertinent information should be typed and turned in. (5 pts.)

3. Students may visit a local, county, or state health agency for the purpose of explaining the role of the agency. A brief report to the class is required. (3 pts.)

4. Students may visit any health agency or health related agency to get printed material for distribution to the class. (2 pts.)

5. Students may bring a cassette, record, or other audio-visual material to class that pertains to the subject under class discussion. All arrangements for the presentation must be made with the instructor one week prior to the presentation. (4 pts.)

6. Students may review a film, cassette, videotape, or other media production from the Triton College Learning Resource Center collection. The student must make all the arrangements to review the material and submit a one page summary of the material in proper manuscript style. (5 pts.)

7. Students may make arrangements to have a guest speaker come to class to discuss the subject under study. Prior approval must be granted a minimum of one week in advance of the presentation. The student will introduce the speaker. (5 pts.)

8. Students may arrange an interview with some person involved in health care service. A written summary of the interview with appropriate data must be turned in prior to the coverage of the material in class. (5 pts.)

9. Students may make an oral report of an interview with some person involved in the health care delivery industry. This material must be useful to class discussion and approved by the instructor. (3 pts.)

10. A student may submit a proposal for extra credit to the instructor. All proposals must be approved a minimum of two weeks prior to the due date. Point totals will range from 1-5. Suggestions for extra credit are: review a book, movie, play, or meeting; attend a seminar or clinic; critique a popular record or tape, a television program on a health related subject; visit a nursing home, mental hospital; or send for health information which would benefit the class or the person.

The handout has been of immense help in answering questions and assigning extra credit projects. Since my work is at the community college level, these activities attract student involvement. Perhaps you might desire to adapt the guidelines to your school environment but my experience has been an increase of interest in extra credit.

Promoting Experiential Learning

MICHAEL HAMRICK is associate professor and head, Division of Health Science and Safety Education, Memphis State University and CAROLYN STONE is patient education coordinator, City of Memphis Hospital, 860 Madison Avenue, Memphis, Tennessee 38103.

Getting students involved in health education experiences outside the classroom—experiential learning—continues to be a pressing need in health education. The purpose of this article is to promote experiential learning in health education by providing a list of projects to encourage out-of-the-classroom learning. While this list was developed for use in the personal health course, similar lists can easily be developed and implemented in courses where it is important to broaden students' experiences and to facilitate awareness of attitudes, behaviors, and lifestyles that are difficult to accomplish in the classroom.

These projects are designed for the student, not the teacher. Therefore, we suggest that the list be duplicated and distributed to students. These projects should be structured into course requirements so that points or some kind of credit can be earned. Since the projects vary in the amount of time, effort, and involvement required, possible points/credits should also vary. Some projects require several months to finish while others may be completed in a 30 minute interview. Students should be encouraged to pursue areas of personal interest and to take advantage of their talents. Some projects require skill in journalism, photography, movie production, art, research, etc. Students should be encouraged to select only those projects which offer a new experience for them. Finally, guidelines should be developed which specify how and when projects are to be reported.

Experiential Learning Projects

1. Do a film. Compile either an 8mm film or 35mm slides focusing on some topic. This display can be incorporated into a multimedia presentation using audio-tape or any other appropriate media. For example, you might produce a tape-slide show on eating habits of college students, study habits, recreational habits, dating habits, marriage from the woman's point of view, people trying to make conversation, children's ideas about death, etc.

2. Prepare an audio-tape collage. Tape many songs, poems, readings or sounds around a particular theme. The theme might be aging, drugs, self-identity, or sexuality.

3. Select one of the health habits/behaviors that you are concerned about and would like to work on. Develop a plan of action which focuses on the desired behavioral change. Use a behavioral modification plan as described in class. Keep a log on the success/failure of the plan. Follow up with an analysis of the plan and the behavior and what you learned.

4. Pair up with someone else to form a health "therapy" dyad. The purpose of the partnership is to have someone with whom the health habit/behavior can be discussed. Meet with your partner several hours a week. See if you can develop a plan for achieving desired behavioral change. Keep a log of your meetings. Use your partner both as a sounding board and as a monitor to keep you honest.

5. During the semester, keep a log of the behaviors/habits you change or modify. Examine the circumstances of the changes. Can you identify a pattern to the changes made? What did you learn? Report results.

6. Keep a journal. Record reactions to occurrences related to some topic or activity. The journal could chronicle a physical fitness regime or dietary pattern or an encounter group experience running throughout the semester.

7. Prepare and implement a research proposal. Some of you may have ideas for experiments such as the effects of various quantities of alcoholic beverages on reaction time, food tasting experiment, survey of attitudes.

8. Conduct a health demonstration. Some topics may lend themselves to a demonstration—the effects of smoking on heart rate, blood pressure, body temperature or how a medical test such as EEG or EKG works and what it shows.

9. Go to the Health Department, Venereal Disease Clinic as if you were a client seeking help for V.D. You may use a false name if you prefer. Report what you learned. How were you treated? What did you observe in the waiting room, the treatment rooms? How did you feel? What changes would you suggest to make the experience less negative for those who need their services?

10. Interview a person or persons who smoke heavily (yourself if you fit the category). Get a profile on their smoking habits, when they smoke, for how long, how it affects them, why they think they smoke, comments of family and friends about the smoker. Have they ever quit? Why? Why did they resume smoking?

11. Go to a setting unfamiliar to your lifestyle and report your reactions, feelings, etc. Try a walk through an inner city neighborhood, attend church services of a different religious group, go to an adult movie or bookstore, a gay bar, or shop at a small country store.

12. Spend an evening in a local hospital's intensive care waiting room. Listen, observe. If you feel comfortable, talk with the families waiting. Record your reactions, what you learned medically as well as emotionally.

13. Spend a morning making rounds with a public health nurse, food sanitation inspector, rat control investigator, or environmentalist.

14. Go to a community health center and take a seat in line. Examine the attitudes of the staff who work there. Talk to some of the patients. Find out how adequate they think their health care is, what problems they have getting to see a doctor, etc.

15. Conduct a health campaign. Select a health topic and conduct an educational campaign such as anti-smoking, hypertension, sickle cell anemia, cervical cancer detection, population control, human relations.

16. Visit a health foods store and make a list of what you see. Interview personnel who work there about their philosophies on eating. Compare prices of similar foods in grocery stores or pharmacies.

17. Spend one weekend evening sitting in a public hospital's emergency room waiting area. The same evening, spend the same amount of time in a private hospital's E.R. Compare the two physical surroundings, personal attitudes of the staff, the patients you see, their families. How comfortable/uncomfortable would you be if you were a patient?

18. Write a letter to a newspaper or magazine about a current health-related issue that really gets your dander up. Turn in a carbon copy.

19. Visit a health spa. What practices seem valid? What claims are made which seem unrealistic, unhealthy, deceptive, evasive? What do you get for how much money?

20. Go to a free lecture on transcendental meditation. How do you think it works? What are the benefits claimed? What sort of impression did you get from the whole experience?

21. Talk with relatives who have planned a funeral. What were their impressions of the funeral business and the people who assisted them? What details must be attended to when planning a funeral? What legal problems did they run into?

22. Find out resources for contraceptive information. Make a list and include costs, if any, for the services and/or the contraceptive materials. List at least ten resources.

23. Go to the local Unemployment Offices. Sit in the waiting room and listen to the talk around you. Describe the place. Read the notices on the board. Describe any contact with the employees. Wear old clothes. As a variation two people can go together, one dressed in old clothes and one in really good clothes. Describe how individuals differed in their reactions to you.

24. Go to any of the pregnancy counseling resources and ask to have a free pregnancy test. Describe the place, the people, how they treated you. If you are male, you can carry in a urine sample saying it is for your girl friend.

25. On a given night watch TV programs during prime time hours and count the incidents which exploit sex, race, religion, minority groups, occupations, etc.

26. Look in the want ads for jobs which routinely hire only men or women. Call and inquire about the job if you are of the opposite sex. What attitudes did you perceive? Quote any remarks made about sex requirements for the job. Sex discrimination is now against the law in hiring practices. Variaton: Work with a person of the opposite sex. Both call and inquire about the job and record the results.

27. Interview a relative or family friend who is retired. Find out how they spend their time, what they like about being retired, what they dislike. What attitudes about being considered "old" do you pick up on?

28. Arrange for the class to "interview" you about a life crisis you have experienced such as divorce, marriage, childbirth, etc. You do not have to answer any question you don't want to. State any limitations before the interview begins.

29. Read an article in a health journal which interests you. Write a two page typed review of the major points of the article. Include your opinion.

30. Survey 5 "lay" magazines (*McCalls, Ladies Home Journal*, etc.) and write a description of the ads which contradict good health practices. You might want to look at magazines such as *Cosmopolitan, Playboy, Oui*, which emphasize attractiveness and appeal. Include a synopsis of the ads' underlying messages.

31. Attend lecture of guest speakers invited to a local university to discuss their views of health related topics. Example: Life after Life lecture, rape prevention demonstration. Summarize the presentation.

32. Attend health education meetings, fairs, programs sponsored by various community agencies. Summarize presentation.

33. Send in health assessment from back of textbook. Summarize what you learned about your health status, risks and behaviors. Takes about 4–6 weeks to get it back.

34. Get a test for diabetes through the Health Department mobile unit, or get a Pap test. Bring the results to class with a written report of how it was done. Ask questions of the personnel as they perform the tests. Try to find out how many people are detected through this system.

35. Write a summary report on the relationship between personality, emotional state, and cancer (see *Psychology Today*, June 1976).

36. Using a very large map of your city, designate the distribution of doctors in the city. Which areas are heavily populated? Which have only a few? Which are undersupplied? You might want to use colored pins to designate different types of physicians. Do the same with dentists. Write your recommendations.

37. Bring an advertisement to class. List its claims. Analyze it for emotional appeal. Are its claims supported by facts? In what ways is the advertisement misleading? Deceiving?

38. From the list of health products investigated by *Consumer Reports* and published in *The Medicine Show*, select one and summarize the findings of *Consumer Reports*. Does the product render any medical or health benefit? What conditions, if any, must be met in its use? What brands are recommended by Consumer Union?

39. Refer to the magazine, *FDA Papers*, a monthly publication of the Food and Drug Administration and identify an example of quackery. What is the claim of the product? What does the FDA say about the product?

Some examples include Weight-away Belt (Feb. '72); LaVive Body Creme (Nov., '70); Paradise Grapefruit Diet (Aug., '71).

40. Tape a radio or TV commercial and bring to class. What kind of propaganda strategy was used? How is it misleading?

41. Conduct a demonstration to test commercial claims of a health product.

42. Write a company for verification of claims made in advertising. Turn in carbon copy of letter and indicate company's response.

43. Write a brief summary report on the published article on chiropractics (See *Consumer Reports*, Sept., Oct., 1975). Write a report on any other health related article included in the monthly publication of *Consumer Reports*.

44. Tell about the decisions a heart attack victim or cancer victim makes in going through treatment, surgery, rehabilitation. Comment on length of stay, financial aspects, steps in rehabilitation, changes in lifestyles, etc.

45. Write a summary report on an article published during the past calendar year on a disease. Compare the information with that in the text and comment on the differences.

46. Develop a skit or role playing situation illustrating some attitudinal or behavioral aspect of a disease. For example, simulate the typical reaction of a person observing a diabetic in insulin shock; the reaction of someone to the news that he or she has a chronic disease.

47. Write a position statement on some controversial aspect of various diseases and be prepared to read to class. The position does not necessarily have to be your own.
A. Epileptics should have limited driving privileges.
B. Medical science is going too far with heart transplants.
C. Government restrictions in the form of laws, penalties should be imposed on persons with genetically related diseases.
D. Marijuana should be legalized for use by glaucoma victims.
E. The government is restricting distribution of laetrile because of loss of profits and government grants in research.

48. Interview a person who by nature of his/her job observes death and dying (police officer, mortician, war veteran, physician, nurse).

49. Develop a skit or role playing situation illustrating some aspect of death. For example, how people act at a funeral home, a family making funeral arrangements.

50. Write a position statement on some controversial aspect of death and dying.
A. Too much money is spent on funerals.
B. Young children should be taken to funerals.
C. Being dead is more honorable than being invalid.
D. Burying bodies is a waste of good, productive land.
E. There is too much death in movies and on TV.

51. Visit an Alcoholics Anonymous meeting and report your experience.

52. Write one page position statement expressing an extreme point of view on alcohol. The position does not have to be your own. Read to class, time permitting.

53. Conduct a genetic experiment in class demonstrating dominant-recessive traits. For example, obtain small crystals of phenylthiocarbamide or PTC test papers. Conduct a taste experiment distinguishing between bitter tasters and non-tasters. What are the expected results?

54. Write a case history or biographical sketch on a person with a genetically related disease or condition. Describe the lifestyle of the person and how it differs from "normality." Describe the effects on the family.

55. Find out what kind of genetic services and counseling are available locally, the conditions for service, prerequisites, costs, location, etc. Report to class.

56. Take a copy of the state penal code from the library and extract the basic criminal statutes relating to sex offenses. Note particularly those describing such acts as rape, seduction, carnal abuse, cohabitation, adultery, indecent exposure, loitering, molesting, and vagrancy. Notice, too, laws relating to marriage, (consent, ceremony, verification) contraceptives, pregnancy, abortion, and venereal disease. Report to class.

57. Develop a skit or role playing situation on some aspect of sexuality or sexually related behavior.

58. Select two newspapers (only one from your city), observe and record for one week the newspapers' statistics on marriages, divorces, and annulment. Graph the results. Include in the graph a breakdown on grounds for divorce.

59. Construct a sample marriage contract for yourself with provisions for facets of marital life you consider particularly important. You may want to consider some of the more common features found in marriage contracts today.
A. division of assets held prior to marriage
B. division of income after marriage

C. to have or not have children
D. responsibilities of partners in child care
E. obligations and rights regarding separate careers

60. Conduct a survey on some aspect of sexuality. For example, married couples of different ages could be asked to answer the following questions.
A. What do you see as the purpose of marriage?
B. Who controls the finances in your family?
C. What effect has the women's movement had on marriage today?
D. What are your views on early marriage?

61. Write a story in the "true confession" style that deals with issues of reproduction, birth control, marriage, parenthood, sex roles, etc. The story may be discussed in class.

62. Write a position paper on one of the following statements.
A. A couple should be encouraged to choose the sex of their baby
B. A single person or gay couple should be allowed to raise a child.
C. Men should assume the responsibility of birth control
D. No one should have more than two children
E. Marriage contracts should become the form of marriage law
F. A couple with hereditary disease should not have children
F. Abortion on demand is a basic human right
H. Unlimited availability of contraceptives encourages promiscuity

63. Conduct an experiment/demonstration in class which focuses on the effects of air pollution, water pollution or noise pollution.

64. Draw a cartoon series which illustrates any health-related topic for example:
A. transmission of venereal disease
B. use of contraceptives
C. access to medical care/physician
D. medical terminology or technology
Design it to get a point across to college level students.

65. Demonstrate in class how to test for blood type; how to test for sugar in urine; pregnancy test; T.B. skin test; test for sickle cell anemia. Be sure you understand the whys and hows of what you are testing for and not just the procedure itself.

66. Interview several women who have experienced menopause. What were their attitudes about it before they experienced it? After they experienced it? What myths about menopause were true/untrue for them? How did it affect their families, their marital relationship? Was any medical treatment given? What were the attitudes of their physicians?

67. Attend a meeting of the LaLeche League, the organization that helps women breast-feed their children. Record what you saw, heard, learned.

68. Compare costs of 15 common prescription drugs among several local pharmacies. Include a chain-owned pharmacy, a small neighborhood one, and a hospital-owned pharmacy. Include the attitudes of those you questioned.

69. Compile a list of local psychiatrists. Call and ask for information on: fee scale, training, group or individual therapy, type of therapy (psychoanalysis, primal therapy, gestalt, electroshock, etc.), hospital affiliation.

70. Contact the local organization for wife abuse. What are their findings regarding wife abuse locally, their services, future plans?

71. Interview someone who lives in what would be considered an alternative lifestyle: communal setting, couple who chooses not to have children, unmarried couple living together, homosexual couple living together. Question each person involved.

72. Collect drawings/paintings from young, preschool children depicting their impressions of sexuality. *Check with parents first!* These could include their concept of anatomy, birth, sex roles, etc. Show these to class with your observations and comments made by children. If you have small children you may use their artwork.

73. Write a report on some new medical "gadget," such as mammography, CAT scanners, fetal monitoring. Include any criticism the technique has received as well as its benefits.

74. Interview a couple who has experienced "natural childbirth" (the Lamaze method).

75. Write a self-help guide to common vaginal infections. Include symptoms, treatment, preventive measures, if any. Alternative topic: insomnia, urinary tract infections.

76. Give blood at one of the hospital blood banks. Bring proof of the donation. Include written report of how community blood donation plan works.

77. Visit a Weight Watchers meeting. Record your experiences along with a description of their program. Include a description of "case histories" you might overhear or learn about. How does their plan work?

78. Write an analysis of migraine headaches: what causes them, what happens when they occur, treatment, new ideas of therapy.

79. Interview an acupuncturist or an osteopath. Thoroughly document their training programs and the usefulness of their skills.

80. Put together a first aid kit designed for a specific purpose (camping, boat, workroom, etc.). Bring to class and explain whys of the contents you chose.

81. Find out and record 20 people's views on raising the mandatory retirement age to 70. Choose a mixture of ages for your subjects.

82. Design a sensitivity exercise to help a group such as a new class break down initial barriers of discomfort. The aims should be to decrease tension about being in a new, strange group and increasing knowledge about each other. Include factors such as: time needed, materials needed, goals, facilitators' roles and responsibilities.

83. Collect at least five health pamphlets from community sources and critique them as to their usefulness, their appeal. Redesign them to make them more "zingy," more appealing.

84. Review filmstrip/tape on one of three consumer products (shampoo, acne treatments, aspirin) and write a critique of it. Include at least five ads for the product which make misleading statements.

85. Take the results of the health knowledge pretest which was administered in class and complete a profile sheet and validation exercise. (See Hamrick, Michael. *Health Education*, Nov.-Dec. 1978, pp. 32-34 for complete instructions).

86. Preview health related films available at local libraries and community agencies. Write a summary report.

87. If none of these projects grab you, think of another. Write a plan of action and turn in for approval. Points will be given after reading project description.

The Hospital as Motivator for Health Learning

Saul Ross is assistant professor of physical education, School of Physical Education and Recreation, University of Ottawa, Ottawa, Canada. Previously he was a teacher and physical education department head at Outremont High School in Montreal, Quebec, and instructor of health and physical education at the High School of Commerce in Ottawa, Ontario.

The problem confronting me was written clearly in the faces of the ninth grade boys staring up at me from behind their desks. A number of factors were operating to produce those defiant looks. Some of the boys were repeating grade 9, and almost everyone in the class had repeated one or two school years previously, either in elementary school or in junior high school. The ages of the pupils ranged from 13 years to 17 years. Their attitude also reflected the low status of health education, confirmed by the fact that it was assigned only one period per week. The low opinion they had was also the result of some prosaic standardized teaching approaches to this subject in their previous schooling.

The challenge was obvious. How could we change their attitude to health education? How would we create interest and excitement? What new method could we find that would involve the students directly? What new area of the curriculum could we investigate that would meet the following criteria: not covered before in previous grades, interesting to all the boys, and something to which they could all relate readily?

Before relating how the challenge was met, it is important to describe the school setting. The High School of Commerce is a beautiful new building, constructed as part of an urban renewal project to meet the needs of the people in the immediate area. It is situated in a low-income, inner city area, amid government office buildings, and close to a large area that has been scheduled for urban redevelopment for some time now. Because the curriculum is geared to commercial subjects, over 75% of the student population is female. Few of the students aspire to university; most hope to land a good job after graduating from high school, fairly confident that the commercial education they received will qualify them for many office jobs. The boys aspire to jobs as office clerks, retail salesmen, management trainees, or junior positions in advertising departments; some hope to join the police force.

My first step was to find out what parts of the health education curriculum had been covered. Each boy was invited to tell me and his classmates what areas he had studied or what he could recall from previous years. The topics mentioned were numerous, and the interest in each one varied. considerably. There did not seem to be a clear pattern, nor an exact core of subjects covered, and this assessment applied equally to both my classes.

Pondering the problem, it occurred to me that one area had been omitted completely; it was an area not covered in the textbooks used for health education. The hospital—the largest, most visible health institution—was a topic ignored completely in their health education courses.

My next problem was how to present this topic to really motivate the students. One entire class period was devoted to having each boy relate his experience with a hospital, be it a visit to a friend or relative, a stay in the hospital, or contact with the institution through service in the emergency department or in one of the clinics. The fears, misconceptions, and negative feelings that emerged confirmed my thinking about the importance of delving into this area.

After every pupil had talked, I asked them to write as many questions as they could think up about hospitals. This was something new to them, and after a few protests about not being able to think up any questions, they set to work. Each student was asked to prepare a list of 15 questions for the next lesson. The assignment seemed tough, but the interest was there.

Plans for the next lesson called for dividing the class into small groups of 4 or 5 boys. Each group selected its own chairman and then set about the task of analyzing the lists of questions to consolidate them into one questionnaire. Questions could be combined and, as discussion took place, new questions were added. Each class handed me 5 question sheets, a process that lasted for two lessons. The questionnaires were mimeographed, with adequate space for answers, ready for use well before our trip to the Ottawa Civic Hospital.

I contacted the Ottawa Civic Hospital and arranged for both classes to have a tour of the hospital. Copies of the questionnaires were sent to the Hospital, to help the people there in planning our tour. The Hospital had never had such a large group (25-30 boys) take a tour, and so they planned an itinerary to take into account the large number as well as the interest of the group as indicated by our questionnaire.

Arrangements were made with the school office to free the classes for the afternoon. The cost of transportation was paid by the travel budget of the Physical and Health Education Department.

The tour included visiting the admissions office, records office, emergency department, furnace and boiler rooms, laundry, kitchen, repair rooms, storage room, and underground passageways. Because of the large numbers of boys, laboratories and wards were omitted. The tour ended in a lecture theater where we heard two speakers. The head nurse of radiology explained the use of X-rays and showed one of a clearly visible fracture. The supervisor of orderlies explained the functions of an orderly and detailed the training program he underwent. Each pupil had a questionnaire with him as we toured the hospital and busily wrote answers as they were provided by our guide. At the end of the tour the boys made their own way home from the hospital.

The next few lessons were devoted to following up what we had learned. The discussions that were held pertaining to the various functions of the hospital indicated that students had gained new insights and attitudes. Heart transplants was a subject of current interest and provided us with a natural and logical lead-in to the next topic—study of the heart and circulatory system.

In reviewing this unit in our health education course, I felt the challenge had been well met. The students were involved. They made up a questionnaire, which truly indicated what they wanted to know. By using the small group process to promote interaction, more questions appeared than with a simple compilation of all the original questions. Interest was high and was sustained during the creation of the questionnaire and during the actual visit. There was considerable excitement about visiting the hospital and being guided on a special tour. The interest reflected a real need. The boys explored a new world on the tour of the hospital, a world few people in the community had seen or even thought about.

Two important questions need to be asked. Did students learn? What did they learn? They certainly learned about the operation of a hospital and became aware of parts of the hospital that most people don't know exist. This new knowledge gave them new insight into the complexity of the institution and made them aware of many new employment categories. They were afforded an opportunity to look into a world unto itself, a complex and vital institution in our community. This new knowledge led to understanding which in turn helped to change the negative feelings the boys had to the institution. Career possibilities in the hospital, specifically the position of an orderly, was important new information. Incidentally, the tour also pointed out to the hospital staff the need to embark on an educational and public relations program designed to modify the feelings of people in the community about the hospital.

While attitude is difficult to measure, and certainly no scientific effort was made to assess this area, I sensed a new interest in health education on the part of the students. By using this experience to launch the next topic—heart and circulatory system—the progression was natural and logical as compared to previous years where new subjects were introduced artificially, merely because they were listed next on the course of study.

Did they learn? What did they learn? By forming the questions they learned about the thing they wanted to know, pinpointing the areas they were most interested in. By constructing the questionnaire, they learned to evaluate and discriminate. Perhaps most important, they were directly involved in the entire process.

Field Trips

JAMES H. PRICE is associate professor of Allied Health Sciences at Kent State University, Kent, Ohio 44240.

Even though field trips are "old" teaching techniques, there are thousands of teachers who never leave the classroom. The community is filled with health resources, and all health teachers should make a list of agencies and places to visit which are related to health education.

The major objective of a field trip is to give students firsthand and accurate experiences not obtainable in the classroom. Trips should be taken only when they can contribute to the objectives of the course. The following questions should be answered before the field trip is planned. Will the students be genuinely interested in the trip? Will certain concepts be more clearly understood as a result of the trip? Will the time and trouble be worth the amount of learning produced? Is the trip truly representative of the unit objectives?

Preliminary planning for a field trip takes considerable work and should be scheduled well in advance of the trip. Anytime the class goes exploring in the community there is the possibility of accidents, but careful planning with attention to details can help eliminate many of the hazards of a field trip. Properly supervised field trips, authorized by the appropriate school authorities, usually involve the same legal liability conditions as any classroom activity. Teachers should find out if their state has special restrictions. Both administrative and parental permission will need to be obtained. The parents' permission slip should identify the who, what, when, where, and why of the field trip and clarify who is legally responsible for insurance coverage of the student.

The teacher should visit the site prior to the trip and plan the observations and activities that will best contribute to the unit objectives. Be sure that restrooms, eating accommodations, and first aid stations have been identified. The development of a route map with points of interest marked can help in-crease learning on the field trip. Arrangements for chaperones, transportation, and finances must be made well in advance of the trip.

Prepare the students for the trip by reviewing the objectives for taking the trip, giving appropriate background information, identifying specific questions

the students should seek answers for, reviewing standards of conduct and safety for traveling and while at the site, identifying any possible allergens or special problems students might encounter (poison ivy, for example). Inform students of special needs, such as clothing, notebooks, expenses, lunch, etc.

Teachers should take along a first aid kit if the trip is going to be all day or if the visitation site does not have first aid supplies. Other items for consideration to take along on the trip include: plastic bags in case someone gets carsick and bags for waste disposal (especially if the students take their lunches).

The group should be kept to a manageable size, by either limiting the number of students who can go or by increasing the number of chaperones and making subgroups. Take along a list of names of all students on the trip and count heads frequently. Other aids are to assign partners for the trip and select a place to meet if a student gets lost. Above all—don't panic! The trip will require a teacher who is enthusiastic, alert, and *flexible*!

Upon arriving at the site, if you are to have a guide, introduce him or her and get the group moving along as quickly as possible. Try to stick to the time schedule while still answering all the students' questions. When leaving, check the class list, thank the guide, and depart promptly. If a problem should arise which will cause the group to be late, telephone the school and let the principal know. This reduces the anxiety in principals and parents who may be waiting for the returning students.

Plan for followup activities after the field trip. Some of the most important learning will come from sharing impressions and discussing events which occurred on the field trip. Further reading, writing, and class projects could grow out of the well-planned field trip. Followup classroom activities will likely reveal to what extent your field trip objectives were met. The class and/or the teacher should follow up and write a thank you letter to the visitation site. A final evaluation of the trip should be formally written and put on file in the main office. Then when other teachers consider visiting the same site, they will have an objective evaluation by one of their colleagues.

HEALTH GAMES

A recent publication presents learning games in several health education content areas.[1] A drug game and an alcohol game from that source are presented here.

What's On My Back

Slang terms for "street drugs" are commonly used. However, the actual drug, its action, its effect, and correct name are often not known. This game will familiarize students with the names, the type, and the effects of drugs. Index cards, felt tip pen and prizes are used. Place a slang term, correct name, and long term effect on separate cards using the list shown here.

Description for Playing: Pin one card on the back of each student without them seeing it.

Instruct the students that they must go to other students and ask for a clue as to

without a doctor's prescription?

Drinking

Alcohol consumption is a widespread practice among all age groups. Alcohol education is one means of correcting the misconceptions many people currently believe and/or practice. This game is designed to help students discriminate between fact and fallacy about drinking.

Description for Playing: One story is given to each student. Intertwined in this story are misconceptions and/or false statements. Each sentence begins with a number. Circle the number of those statements which are *not* true.

Name	Slang Name	Effect
Amphetamines	bennies, dexies, pep pills, uppers, hearts	Alertness, actively paranoid, loss of appetite, delusions, hallucinations.
Barbiturates	barbs, blue devils, downers	Euphoria, physical dependency with dangerous withdrawal symptoms.
Cocaine	coke, snow, snuff	Excitation, sore nose, paranoia, depressive rebound on withdrawal.
Codeine		Euphoria, physical dependence, constipation, loss of appetite.
Heroin	H., horse, scat, junk, smack, hard stuff	Euphoria, physical dependence, constipation, loss of appetite.
LSD	acid, sugar, sunshine	Insightful experiences, distortion of senses, may intensify existing psychosis, panic reactions, "flashbacks."
Marijuana	pot, grass, tea, MJ, weed	Outside stimuli more vivid, relaxation, euphoria, physical dependence.
Methadone	meth	Constipation, loss of appetite.
Morphine	white stuff, morph	Euphoria, physical dependence, constipation, loss of appetite.

"What's on my back" such as an effect, drug name, or slang term.

After a person correctly guesses what his card says he then finds the other students with the rest of the information pertaining to a certain drug. The first group with the correct cards wins a prize.

Discussion Question: 1. What are the immediate effects of each drug?

2. What are stimulants, depressants or hallucinogens?

3. What is the legal, social, physical danger of many of these drugs taken

[1]Woody, age 20, resides with his parents in Mt. Pleasant where he is a sophomore at the university. [2]The females on campus find him very attractive; 6 feet tall, 175 pounds, blond curly hair, and bright, blue eyes. [3]Final exam week has brought about the usual stress, and anxiety many college students experience. [4]In an effort to alleviate the stress, Woody attended a weekend party. [5]It was the usual kind of party he attended with a lot of women, booze and loud music. [6]Many of the females at the party were in constant pursuit of him because his ability to drink

more than anyone else was viewed as a sign of virility. [7]This is partly due to the fact that the alcohol he consumed affected his muscles first. [8]In Woody's case, the alcohol also acted as an aphrodisiac, as alcohol consumption usually does. [9]With these two factors contributing to his virility, one can plainly see why he was pursued.

[10]Woody is a fairly bright guy and has established guidelines for his drinking behavior. [11]First, he always drinks vodka to prevent rapid absorption. [12]Second, he seldom eats any food before he drinks because it fills his stomach and he cannot hold as many drinks. [13]After all, if it's free booze he wants to get all he can. [14]Third, he drinks slowly instead of gulping his drinks to prevent getting intoxicated.

[15]Since he is physically a big guy, he really can drink as much as he wants because he has more body tissue and fluids to dilute the alcohol.

[16]As the evening progressed (3 hours), Woody consumed six mixed drinks (1½ oz. alcohol per drink) and the only observable sign he showed was a slight intensification of his talkative personality.

[17]As the party continued, he talked with friends, danced and asked Joey, an attractive girl clad in jeans, if he could drive her home. [18]Of course, Joey answered yes, and they left the party.

[19]Should Joey have more carefully considered the possible consequences of leaving with Woody? [20]After all, he was only drinking moderately and there are no risks if he drinks moderately. [21]He wasn't acting "funny;" the alcohol he drank stimulated him—that's the primary effect it has on a person. [22]And because both his parents are alcoholics he probably has inherited alcoholism from them. [23]Oh well, why should she worry?

[24]The simple truth of this story is that Joey is the alcoholic and not Woody. [25]Everyone knows that there are more women alcoholics than men.

Questions: Which statements are false? (6, 7, 8, 11, 12, 15, 16, 20, 21, 22, 25).

Important Considerations: The instructor should carefully explain why the above statements are incorrect. This exercise can be used as a pretest prior to discussion or as an evaluative tool after discussion.

[1]Ruth C. Engs, ed., Eugene Barnes, and Molly Wantz, *Health Games Students Play* (Indiana University: Bloomington, Indiana, 1974), pp. 13-23.

Health Games, Simulations, and Activities

DAVID E. CORBIN is in the School of HPER, University of Nebraska, Omaha, Nebraska 68182 and DAVID A. SLEET is director of the Center for Health Games and Simulations, College of Human Services, San Diego State University, San Diego, California 92182.

Games and simulations are widely used as teaching aids by classroom teachers across the country. We think this attests to the potential of simulation and gaming activities in instruction. The Center for Health Games and Simulations at San Diego State University houses the largest single collection of health games and simulations and serves as a resource center for these materials.

During the past five years, we have collected, cataloged, and evaluated games in health for the benefit of consumers. We have found that materials vary enormously in content, complexity, and price—ranging from one-to-one patient education games for under $5.00, to computerized simulators for over $500.00.

The purpose of this article is to give examples of games which can be conducted with little cost or preparation time. After experimenting with these suggestions, you can decide if you want to pursue more formal and expensive commercial products.

Drug Knowledge Game

Print the names of different drugs on index cards, one per student. Be certain to use terms that are appropriate for the grade level you are teaching. See the following examples. Notice that group names, brand names, generic names, and common names are used.

Elementary	Middle School
cough syrup	marijuana
aspirin	nicotine
beer	caffeine
tobacco	glue
coffee	antacids
Tums	Nytol
Rolaids	Sominex
	whiskey
	Anacin
	milk of magnesia

High School	Post High School
heroin	psilocybin
codeine	penicillin
LSD	THC
gin	methadone
Midol	Valium
Ex-lax	Librium
Contact	hallucinogens
hashish	methedrine
wine	peyote
Bufferin	alcohol
cocaine	nitrous oxide
opium	PCP
	morphine
	amphetamines
	mescaline

Next, pin a drug card on the back of each student making sure the student does not know what is written on the card. The object of the game is for students to guess the name of the drug or drug group pinned on their own backs by asking questions of fellow students. Students should stand up and mingle in a cleared area of the classroom.

The rules are as follows.

1. Ask only yes or no questions.

2. Limit questions to three per person. This forces students to seek information from people other than their friends.

3. Approach the game cooperatively not competitively. Once a person guesses his or her own drug card, pin the card to the lapel. That student continues to mingle answering questions for other students. If time is a problem, set a limit.

Variation: Once the drug is guessed, pin a second card to the student's back for the student to guess.

Use: This game can illustrate how much or how little students know about drugs. Students will find they have been given conflicting information. It will also show some of the problems encountered in the drug culture; for example, buying drugs on the street is not very reliable. A drug may be substituted for another without the buyer's knowledge. Sometimes the seller does not know the difference between drugs. This game can help reinforce the idea that peers are not always reliable sources of information, nor are the sellers of drugs.

This game can also help improve questioning skills and reasoning. If the questions start out general and then become increasingly specific, students will be more successful in guessing their cards. Here are some sample questions—Am I an upper? Am I legal? Am I injected?

Drug Grouping Game

This game is adapted from the game, "Birds, Beasts, and Fowl," by George Enell, Kay Hardman, and Noreen Dresser (1977). It can be used as an offshoot of the drug knowledge game or on its own.

With a drug name card pinned to their lapels, students group themselves according to their cards without talking to each other. The teacher should not tell the students how to group themselves at this point.

After the students have settled into groups, one student from each group leaves the room. The teacher now asks members of different groups what their group is. After they are in agreement, the person outside the room returns and gives his or her perception of the group to see if it is the same as that of the rest of the group.

After this exercise is over you can give more specific instructions for the next segment. For example: Group yourselves into two categories—legal and illegal; or five groups—stimulants, depressants, hallucinogens, narcotics, and others. You can experiment with many possibilities, all of which will help the students learn about drugs and various classifications.

After each grouping exercise, check to make sure all students are in the proper group. If they are not, ask the class if they can find the person or persons who should change groups. Some can fit into more than one group, for example if the groups are legal and illegal then barbiturates could be in either, since they can be prescribed or sold illegally.

Remember, students may not talk while grouping themselves, they must rely on reading the drug cards and "body language" to determine where they belong.

Reproductive System Terms Game

This game is played in exactly the same manner as the drug knowledge game only cards with names of the male and female reproductive system parts are pinned on the backs of the students. This is an excellent activity *for teachers* who will be teaching sex education, since it helps them to talk freely and openly about terms having to do with reproduction. It is not recommended for generalized audiences. Like the drug knowledge game, it helps to illustrate the misinformation that abounds among peers.

Cards can include any of the following

hymen	labia majora
testes	Bartholin's glands
epididymus	urethra
seminal vesicles	glans
fallopian tubes	labia minora
ovaries	Graafian follicle
foreskin	cervix
uterus	clitoris
prostate	seminiferous
vas deferens	tubules
	vagina
bulbourethral or Cowper's glands	
penis	

Note: "urethra" is part of the male and female anatomy, but, of course, only in the male's reproductive system—this may make it a more difficult term for some.

Food Grouping Game

This game is very similar to the drug grouping game and is also adapted from "Birds, Beasts, and Fowl." Instead of name tags cut out pictures of different foods from magazines. Be certain that you select different foods from all food groups and pseudo-foods such as alcoholic beverages, salt, pepper, condiments. Place all the pictures into a paper bag then have students remove one food cutout without looking and pin it on their lapels. From this point on, the progression is the same as the drug grouping game. Remember, students always group themselves without talking to each other.

Variations: Ask six people to leave the room. Ask the rest of the class to regroup themselves according to their tags this time according to a specific direction, such as foods high in sugar, a balanced meal, high protein foods. When the other students come back into the room they try to guess upon what basis the groups have been formed.

Ask all students to form the four basic food groups (or the basic seven). Make necessary corrections by asking the class as a whole if everyone is in the correct group. If they don't know, help them.

Ask the students to group into foods that are high-risk for dental disease and foods that are low-risk for dental disease.

Ask the students to group into high-risk, neutral, and low-risk for cardiovascular disease.

Experiment with other groupings. After this exercise, students can easily see that there are many different aspects to consider in selecting foods. Just because a food may be low-risk for dental disease, does not mean it is necessarily low-risk for cardiovascular disease. We also like to add foods such as pizza or hamburger which don't fit neatly into any single group.

"Drunk" Synonym Game

There are, reportedly, more synonyms for the word "drunk" than for any other word in the English language. These words say something about how ingrained and accepted alcohol is in our society. To begin this game open the floor to any and all synonyms for the word "drunk." As the students call them out, write them on the blackboard.

Examples:

juiced	inebriated
plastered	pickled
polluted	under the table
zonked	smashed
blasted	loaded
tight	intoxicated

To better see how our society views drunkenness, make another list in categories. This can be done as a class or as an assignment for each individual. The categories could be: technical-medical, funny-happy, tragic-sad, and neutral. Discuss the implications. Invariably the funny-happy category is the largest.

To extend this activity, students can name plays, movies, comic strips, TV shows, and people in which (or whom) alcohol plays an integral part, then categorize them the same way they did the synonyms.

Examples:

Foster Brooks	"Lady Sings the Blues"
Dean Martin	Betty Ford
Andy Capp	Alice Cooper
Ed McMahon	"Streetcar Named Desire"
Hagar	"All in the Family"
Janis Joplin	"Days of Wine and Roses"
W. C. Fields	Wilbur Mills

After trying any of these games, you may wish to try some of the other games on file at the Center for Health Games and Simulations. For more information on the use of games and simulations in health instruction, the reader is encouraged to consult the suggested readings.

Suggested Readings

1. Sleet, D. A. and Corbin, D. E., "Simulation Gaming in Health Education," in The Handbook of Health Education, P. Lazes, ed. Germantown, MD: Aspen Systems, 1979.

2. Sleet, D. A. and Stadsklev, R., "Annotated Bibliography of Simulations and Games in Health Education," Health Education Monographs, Vol. 5, Supplement 1, 1977 pp. 74–90.

3. Sleet, D. A. and Bearman, D., Games Patients Play: Simulation and Health Care, Behavioral Medicine, Vol 5 (12) December, 1978, p. 32–37.

4. Engs, R.; Barnes, S. and Wantz, M. Health Games Students Play. Dubuque, IA: Kendall-Hunt, 1975.

5. Sleet, D. A. and Wertz, R. R. "The Relationship of Simulation/Gaming to Learning Outcomes in Nutrition Education," in Nutrition in Transition, P. White and N. Selvey, eds. American Medical Association, 1978, p. 399–400.

6. Louv, R., Games for Health: Special Report. Human Behavior, Vol. 7 (12), December 1978, pp. 48–49.

7. Clark, C. C. Classroom Skills for Nurse Educators. N.Y.: Springer, 1978.

8. Jacobson, R. L. Teaching with Games Chronicle of Higher Education, Nov. 26, 1979.

9. Sleet, D. A. and Hileman, L. Guide to Health Instruction: Simulations, Games and Related Activities. Irvine, CA: Human Behavior Research Group, 1980.

10. Sleet, D. A.; Noto, J.; and Parker, B. The Use of Simulation Gaming in Safety Education. Control (Australia), Vol. 6, No. 1, pp. 17–25. Feb. 1980.

Originally presented at Association for Advancement of Health Education Meeting, New Orleans, LA. March 1979.

LEARNING GAMES

Getting To Know One Another

There are several interesting ways for students to get to know one another better. Even though they are in the same class, some students never converse with or know much about many of their classmates. The following exercise provides for a discussion of content within a process designed to expand communication in the classroom; it thereby also increases a sense of trust among class members.

Each pupil is asked to select another pupil with whom to discuss one of several listed topics. The partner selected, however, should be someone whom the selector doesn't know very well. Before discussing the topic, each pair gets to know each other better by discussing their aspirations, feelings about the class, family history, or other matters personal to their lives. After this discussion is completed, the content topic is discussed. Twenty minutes should be allowed for this phase of the exercise.

Possible topics for discussion are:

Foods that I like to eat. (Nutrition)

How to make our homes safe. (Safety education)

How girls are different from boys. (Sex education)

Next, each pair chooses another pair whom they don't know very well, and the process is repeated. This time, however, each pupil introduces his partner to the other pair and a general discussion of pupil's backgrounds, etc. precedes the content-related discussion. The group of four can then be combined with another group of four to make eights and eights can be combined to make sixteens, etc.

Listening Practice

Students are formed into groups of three for the purpose of discussing a question. Questions may range from "How does someone make friends?" to "What's the safest way to ride a bicycle?" During the ensuing discussion, in order for a member of the group to communicate verbally, that member must paraphrase, to the satisfaction of the previous speaker, what was last said. If a paraphrase is attempted but is incorrect, the person who is being paraphrased repeats what he said and the paraphraser again attempts to paraphrase his comments. The purposes of this exercise are:

1. To provide a framework for classmates to talk in small groups and get to know one another.

2. To emphasize that we are often thinking of what we want to say and not listening to what others are saying.

3. To discuss fully the topic at hand in an interesting and effective manner.

4. To underline that communication is often impeded by emotional involvement in the topic, someone who talks for a long period of time, someone who presents a lot of ideas all at once, serious biases, or a poor facility in which to talk and listen. Any of the above can, and often do, create difficulties in hearing accurately what is being communicated and can cause difficulty in paraphrasing.

If this exercise is conducted for a twenty minute period and then discussed fully, pupils will become aware of their listening skills and attempt to sharpen them. A periodic repeat of this exercise will provide feedback on progress in development of listening skills.

Family Drawings

Often children's insights into their family lives are not such that the roles of the family members are readily accessible to them. Perceptions of family life are often repressed and hidden. An activity designed to bring to the surface a child's feelings about his family is one in which he draws a picture of his family in a group activity or some other context. At the conclusion of this activity, drawings are exchanged among all members of the class until each classmate has had the opportunity to review each drawing. Pupils write a one sentence comment, which expresses their reaction, on the back of each drawing they review. Comments should relate to the family as a whole, or to individuals depicted. Next, drawings are returned to the artists with time provided to read the comments of their classmates. A discussion follows of the objectives of this exercise.

Lost on the Moon

This activity helps children to compromise and take part in consensual decision making processes. Each child is supplied with a copy of the following problem:

You are in a space crew originally scheduled to rendezvous with a mother ship on the lighted surface of the moon. Mechanical difficulties, however, have forced your ship to crash land at a spot some 200 miles from the rendezvous point. The rough landing damaged much of the equipment aboard. Since survival depends on reaching the mother ship, the most critical items available must be chosen for the 200-mile trip. The fifteen items left intact after the landing are listed below. Your task is to rank them in terms of their importance to your crew in its attempt to reach the rendezvous point. Place number 1 by the most important item, number 2 by the second most important, and so on through the least important, number 15.

_____ Box of matches
_____ Food concentrates
_____ 50 feet of nylon rope
_____ Parachute silk
_____ Portable heating unit
_____ Two .45 caliber pistols
_____ One case dehydrated milk
_____ Two 100-pound tanks of oxygen
_____ Stellar map of the moon's constellation
_____ Life raft containing CO_2 bottles
_____ Magnetic compass
_____ 5 gallons of water
_____ Signal flares
_____ First-aid kit containing injection needles
_____ Solar-powered FM receiver-transmitter

Below are the correct rankings as determined by National Aeronautics and Space Administration:

15—Box of matches (little or no use on the moon)

4—Food concentrate (supply daily food required)

6—50 Feet of nylon rope (useful in tying injured, help in climbing)

8—Parachute silk (shelter against sun's rays)

13—Portable heating unit (useful only if party landed on dark side)

11—Two .45 caliber pistols (self-propulsion devices could be made for them)

12—One case dehydrated milk (food, mixed with water for drinking)

1—Two 100-pound tanks of oxygen (fills respiration requirement)

3—Stellar map of the moon's constellation (one of the principal means of finding direction)

9—Life raft (CO_2 bottles for self-propulsion across chasms, etc.)

14—Magnetic compass (probably no magnetized poles; thus useless)

2—5 gallons of water (replenishes loss by sweating, etc.)

10—Signal flares (distress call within line of sight)

7—First-aid kit containing injection needles (oral pills or injection medicine valuable)

5—Solar-powered FM receiver-transmitter (distress signal transmitter, possible communication with mother ship).

Each child ranks the fifteen items in terms of importance. Groups of six to eight students are then formed to rank the fifteen items as a group, utilizing consensual decision making rather than voting. No one group member's opinion is allowed to override the group's decision. A comparison of individual and group opinions evidences the advantage of consensual decision making. This analysis is conducted by computing the difference between the NASA rankings and the individual rankings firstly, and the NASA rankings and the group's rankings secondly. The differences for the individual rankings are totaled, as are the differences for the group rankings. The lower the score, the more accurate the rankings.[1]

Cognitive Football

A football field is drawn on the blackboard, and the class is divided into two teams. A content area in health education is selected, for example, nutrition. The teacher has three sets of cards which contain questions pertaining to the content area selected. One set of cards contains relatively easy questions, which when answered correctly, result in a five-yard gain. Another set of questions, somewhat more difficult, result in a ten-yard gain; and the last set of questions is worth 15 yards. The toss of a coin decides which team begins the game with the ball on the fifty-yard line. Team members decide, previous to attempting to answer the question, from which set of cards the question should be selected and thereby how much of a gain will be attempted. Teams alternate answering questions and the team that puts the ball over the opponents' goal line is the winner. Only one team member is allowed to answer the question and may not receive help from his teammates.

Written Conversations

This activity serves to correlate language arts with health instruction and, in particular, family living. The class is separated into pairs, one person assigned the role of child and the other the role of parent. A situation is described, e.g., the child wants to play outdoors with his friends while the parent insists he stay indoors and complete his homework. Each pair then engages in a written conversation recorded on a sheet of paper. No verbalizing is permitted. These paper and pencil conversations should last approximately twenty minutes at which time pairs volunteer to read their conversations to the class. Each conversation read is analyzed with access to "replays" since the conversation has been recorded on paper.

[1] Gene Stanford and Barbara Stanford, _Learning Discussion Skills Through Games_ (New York: Citation Press, 1969), pp. 44-47.

HORSE RACING IN THE CLASSROOM

PHILLIP HOSSLER is a teacher of health and physical education and trainer for all sports at the Madison Township High School, Old Bridge, New Jersey 08857.

One of the difficult problems faced by high school educators today is motivating their students, especially in required courses. The problem is convincing students that just because they have to be in the class is no reason why they can't enjoy it and learn something at the same time. Giving stars or lollipops for answering a difficult question or solving a problem is not successful in high school, because older students feel their performance deserves a more beneficial reward, such as the improvement of their grade. In many required courses the students may only do that which is required to pass the course. Clearly what is needed is some sort of activity where the older students are able to feel they are properly reimbursed for their endeavors and still learn something in the process.

I initiated an activity in my health classes wherein the students researched, in class, answers to questions and explanations to the notes that I planned to cover that day. This activity took the form of a horse race. To start class when I use the horse race, I blow a whistle or ring a bell. I have signs in the room saying "Stables," "Race Tips," "Cashier," "Grandstand," etc., and have long strings of colored flags hanging in the room to add authenticity and show the class that I too have enthusiasm and enjoy what I am doing.

Each group of four students is a horse, so there are four jockeys to each horse, and each horse has a name. The first day I put on the overhead projector the drawing of the oval track with the grandstands, flags, and finish line drawn in. In the center of the track I wrote "Hossler's Happy Healthy Horse Sweepstakes." Next I showed on the overhead the ideas I planned to cover that day. For example, when the class starts the study of venereal disease, the notes might look like:

    Intro to VD
    Venus
    skin-to-skin contact
    pox, clap
    cause
    damage to infected

Then I give the class 10-15 minutes to look through the books and pamphlets that I have brought to class or ones they have gotten themselves to discover what I mean by each of these short phrases. Each of the horses is questioned to explain my own notes to me. I speak to a different jockey each time so that everyone is involved at some point.

Each of the phrases is worth a certain point value, usually 1 point. If only one horse gives the correct answer, that horse would get the full point; if two horses give me equally correct answers they would each get one-half point and so forth. The points that each horse receives determine its position around the track. It takes a total of 12 points to run the length of the track.

For example, if horse #1, Sugar Daddy, tells me that skin-to-skin contact is the method of transmission when speaking about venereal disease, he would be correct. If no other horse was able to give me this answer Sugar Daddy would receive the full point. If, however, horse #5, Carmel Corn, told me that skin-to-skin contact was the method of transmitting venereal disease and that coitus was the most common form of skin-to-skin contact for transmitting VD, Carmel Corn would receive three-fourths of a point or he might even steal the full point away from Sugar Daddy since Carmel Corn gave me the more complete answer. The students become involved with the race because of the constant advancing and falling behind on each question. After two or three notes, I write the position of the horses on the track. The jockeys then begin to dig a little deeper the next time for that bit of extra information that will give them the edge over the rest of the pack.

I have also found that researching answers develops teamwork and pride among the jockeys on each horse. They must research much material in a short period of time, so the notes are delegated to each of the jockeys on the horse so that one might have the answer to a note that the other jockeys didn't have time to find.

After each horse has given me an answer explaining the note, I write the points awarded on the overhead next to their horse's name amid cheers and groans from the jockeys. Then I tell them exactly what I was looking for and give them time to write it in their notebooks before going on to the next note. The order in which the horses respond varies each time so no one horse gains an advantage by being the last to answer each time.

The race continues until all the horses have finished the course. If horse #1 finished first the jockeys cannot sit back and do nothing; they must still answer questions to ensure that another one of the horses doesn't earn more points and "nose them out at the wire."

If there are six horses running, the jockeys on the winning horse each get six points, the second place jockeys each get five points, and so forth. These bonus points are used at the end of the marking period when grades are determined.

This method of teaching requires more time, because the amount of material covered each day may not be as much as with the lecture method. It requires a teacher who is able to instruct and still maintain control of the class amid mild chaos, much laughter, and student enthusiasm. I have found that the grades on the tests after using this method are the highest grades of the marking period.

I personally enjoy using this method of teaching. I don't use it for the entire marking period; instead I tell the class about it in the beginning and then save it until last. This also helps to build enthusiasm toward the activity.

FANTASY GAMES

RALPH BATES is in the Department of Health, Physical Education and Recreation, Ohio State University, Columbus, Ohio 43210.

I have used fantasy games with young children, older children, and adults and have found them to be very successful. Participants become more aware of how they perceive themselves, what they are like as people, their strengths and weaknesses and, most important, they can become aware of emotions and deeper feelings which normally would not be disclosed to individual or group members. I have also found that fantasy is relaxing, helps develop better listening skills, and leads to closer, more meaningful relationships among participants.

In this paper I would like to share several of these games, to use with groups of children as a means of relaxation and to help them learn more about themselves. I will indicate the method I use in presenting these games, and the reader can adapt each one according to individual needs. The books and articles in the bibliography are excellent resources for fantasy games as well as other communication skills for both children and adults.

Make A Person

I have found this game to be effective with children to help you learn what they are like as people.

1. Ask a group of children to think of a person's name and write it on the board.

2. Using the general background of the group as a guide, and the age of the children you are dealing with, establish same criteria for this person. Example: "Billy is 14 and lives at home with his mother, father, brother, and sister."

3. Ask the children the following: With help from each one of you, I would like to find out more about Billy. What is he like as a person? What is he like at home? How does he do in school? What does he like to do? How does he feel about himself? With these general questions as a guide, obtain several responses from each child and write them on the blackboard. If you listen carefully, you will be surprised about how these children feel about themselves, their peers, and their families. Follow this through with a group discussion.

Rosebush and Object Identification

This game is directed more toward older children. You may use the same format for younger children by substituting a flower or animal for the rosebush and object.

1. Ask the participants to close their eyes and get as comfortable as possible. They may sit in their chairs or sit or lie on the floor. Then say the following: I am going to take you on a fantasy trip. I want you to do exactly as I say and be aware of nothing else but my voice.

2. The following questions can be used for the rosebush. You will have to adapt these questions to the other games. What are you like as a rosebush (object)? What are your roots like . . . your stem . . . your leaves . . . your thorns . . . your flowers? What are your surroundings like? What season?

3. Now proceed with the following: In several minutes I will ask you to open your eyes then tell us what you are like as a rosebush. Have each member select a group member after he has described himself to the group. The following questions may be used for discussion.

1. What did you learn about yourself?
2. What did the group learn?
3. How does this relate to disclosure, listening, feedback, communication, and fantasy? (Adapted from Stevens, *Awareness*.)

Ocean Trip

Obtain a record or tape of ocean sounds such as *Environmental Sounds*, or a tape recording from a radio or TV communication center.

1. Have the group relax at their desks or lie on the floor.

2. Tell them the following: I am going to take you on a fantasy ocean trip. I want you to close your eyes, relax, and concentrate on what I say. Imagine yourself approaching a beautiful vacated beach. . . . You begin to walk in the sand. . . . Stop and take off your shoes. As you stand there, feel the sand on the bottom of your feet, the grains of sand sifting through your toes. . . . become aware of that feeling. Begin a stroll toward the water's edge. . . . As you continue your walk, become aware of the sun beating on your face, smell the salty air, hear all the sounds around you. Find a spot ahead of you and sit down in the sand. . . . Hold some sand in your hand. . . . Feel the individual grains of sand sift through your fingers. Stand up and continue your stroll toward the water's edge. . . . Before you reach the water, stand (and sit) in the wet sand. . . . Feel your feet sink into the wet sand. Grab a handful of wet sand. . . . Be aware of the difference between the wet sand and the dry sand. Stand by the water's edge. . . . Feel the water gently flowing under your feet and around your ankles. . . . Stand there and smell the salty air, feel the wind blowing in your face, and be aware of all the sounds around you. . . . (cont'd) . . . .

Use your own imagination with this game. After you are through give the group several minutes before they open their eyes and disclose their trip to the group.

The following questions may be used for discussion:
1. How was your fantasy trip?
2. Where were you?
3. What were your surroundings like?
4. What were some of the feelings you experienced?
5. Could you feel the different textures of sand?

Fantasy Dream (This exercise is also directed toward older groups of children.)

Close your eyes and become as relaxed as possible. I am going to take you back to your early childhood to a recurring dream that you used to have then, a dream that you are going to have again.

Don't be afraid. Just concentrate on what I will tell you, and on your experience as my words are spoken. At night, while you are asleep as a small child, the dream would occur over and over again. The dream would begin in the same way. You would get out of bed and walk across the bedroom to the closet. There is now a door behind the closet, a door which you could never find while awake. As you approach the door in your dream it now opens.

As you stand in the door you look down an ancient looking stone staircase. In the dim light you begin to descend the staircase, not at all afraid, down a step at a time. As you approach the bottom of the staircase you stop and hear the gentle sound of water lapping against the rocks below. You approach the water's edge. A small boat is tied to the rocks. Sit in the boat and untie it. Just lie back in the bottom of the boat and let it take you where it wants to go. Sit there, relax, and listen to the water lapping against the boat and rocks, as you gently rock back and forth, back and forth, as the boat drifts down the stream.

As you lie there enjoying your trip you notice a small opening ahead of you. As you approach the opening it becomes larger and larger. You come out of the opening into a new environment which you will now experience. Continue to keep your eyes closed and become aware of the new environment. Where are you? . . . What is it like? . . . What will you do next? . . . What sights, odors, sounds, and movements are you now experiencing? . . . etc. . . . Now open your eyes and disclose your experiences to the group. (Adapted from Masters, *Mind Games*.)

Bibliography

Richard DeMille, *Put Your Mother on the Ceiling* (Addison-Wesley: Reading, Massachusetts, 1974).

Joan Freyberg, "Increasing Children's Fantasies," *Psychology Today*, January 1975.

Lucile Herfat, "The Gut-level Needs of Kids," *Learning*, October 1973.

Edmund Jacobson, *Teaching and Learning: New Methods for Old Arts* (National Foundation for Progressive Relaxation: Chicago, 1973).

Dorothy Jameward, *Born to Win* (Addison-Wesley: Reading, Massachusetts, 1973).

Robert Johnson, *Reaching Out* (Prentice-Hall: Englewood Cliffs, New Jersey, 1972).

Howard Lewis, *Growth Games* (Bantam: New York, 1972).

Robert Masters, *Mind Games* (Delta: Van Nuys, California, 1972).

J. William Pfeiffer, *A Handbook of Structural Experiences for Human Relations Training*, vols. I-IV (University Associates: Iowa City, Iowa, 1972).

John O. Stevens, *Awareness* (Library of Congress: Washington, D.C., 1971).

CHOICES

LYNN TEPER-SINGER is an assistant professor in the Department of Health Science, Physical Education, and Guidance and Counseling at Long Island University—the Brooklyn Center, Brooklyn, New York 11201.

One of my beliefs is that the way one feels about oneself is reflected by the choices one makes and the behavior that follows these choices. Therefore, one of the ways I gain an understanding of the individuals within my health classes is by observing their behavior in here and now situations. Then, by exploring the motivations behind their actions, the class takes part in understanding their decisions.

I have found that the following technique arouses strong emotional responses while dealing with making decisions:

Have your class stand in a circle and look around the room at their classmates picking out one person they would like to know better. At a signal from you, their task will be to go over to the person of their choice and nonverbally show that person how they feel. Often no one will move initially. If this occurs you may wait, or you might encourage them further by saying, "You mean no one here wants to know anyone better." This may be met with a display of discomfort or laughter, and at this point it is best to investigate what the students were feeling by discussing their objections to moving. Even if no one in the class responds to the initial experiment, reactions are taking place within each person. Some members may be confused about who they would choose or how they would show their feelings and therefore might not be able to make a decision. They may have thought it over and decided to do nothing. Some people might have hoped that someone would make a decision to come over to them, relieving them of having to initiate the action.

Questions may be raised for classes that will help students tie in their experiences to making choices. The following is one way that this can be explored.

(1) What were your feelings: when I told you what the initial task would be; while you were moving or anticipating someone else's move; after the task was completed?

(2) How did you decide: (a) who you would like to know better; (b) how you would show that person how you feel; (c) whether or not you would act on your feeling?

(3) Outside life experiences in the classroom: (recommended for small groups)

Under what other circumstances have you experienced similar feelings to those you felt here today?

What decisions did you make under those circumstances?

What correlations can you make that will help you understand the patterns of your choices?

What other alternatives do you believe are open to you?

How do you see your ability to make decisions as a reflection of your self image?

During experiences of this sort within classes on both the high school and college level, I have found that it is immaterial whether or not the class moves at your signal. In both cases, students have disclosed feelings about: (1) being rejected—the feeling that the person they choose may not be open to them. (2) Being misunderstood—someone might interpret their action (to the same or opposite sex) as one of sexual interest. (3) Being special—hoping someone would show them their feelings first. (4) Being a risk-taker—in spite of having all the above feelings the person may decide to move.

Some students claim that they like the opportunity to let their feelings be known and are more comfortable showing their feelings than telling someone about them.

This technique is multifaceted. The conflict that takes place within each person often deals with both the feelings the person has about what he wants or doesn't want to do and the feelings about what others want or expect of him. Another area for discussion, therefore, can include what effect other people have on the decision-making process within individuals.

It is my opinion that those teachers who make their own decision to try this technique will find it to be an excellent tool for helping students to discover and understand the decision-making process and their motivations behind the choices they make.

Constructing an Educational Game

SALLY L. EASTERBROOK is an instructor of health education, Department of Health Sciences, Towson State University, Baltimore, Maryland 21204. This article is adapted from a presentation given to the Maryland AAHPER Convention in October 1976, Largo, Maryland.

There are numerous types of games which can be used in a classroom. Among these are the commercially produced game, teacher adapted game, teacher made game, student adapted game, and student made game. The last four are the least expensive. An additional advantage is that they can be constructed to meet specific needs. Steps for developing an educational game for classroom use follow.

1. First, it is essential to know the capabilities of the students who will be using the game—their abilities, attention spans, and reading levels.

2. A prerequisite in game building is to outline clearly the specific purpose of the game. The constructor should know exactly how it will be used in the classroom.

Games can be used: to introduce new topics, which creates a "set" for the learners; to illustrate an idea; or to review a unit. Some games may be used as pretests and then adapted to serve as a posttest at the end of the unit.

3. Once the purpose of the game has been formulated, the specific content can be outlined.

4. The constructor must then answer some questions concerning the classroom atmosphere during the game.

How quiet or disruptive should the game be?
How many students will be directly involved in game play?
If not all students are involved, what can the rest do?
How much competition should be encouraged through use of this particular game?
How much time needs to be set aside for the playing of this game?

5. Next, the constructor needs to decide what type of game to create—a board game, a word game, a team game, or some other format? What types of questions may be open-ended; based on choice, or short answer? Some questions may be opened ended; based on student answers, the players will have to make certain decisions (branching).

6. Actual construction of the game comes next. Parts should be kept to a minimum to prevent the loss and necessary replacement of pieces. If a board game is being constructed, the board should be neat and colorful. All parts should be safe and durable. Covering parts with clear contact paper decreases "wear and tear."

The construction of directions falls into this step also. Directions should be as uncomplicated, clear, and concise as possible. The object of the game should be stated and all possible situations should be included. If questions are asked during the game, an answer booklet providing all acceptable responses should be provided.

7. The last step in game construction is a trial run. A group of students should play the game on their own. From observations made during this session, modifications of time requirements, rules, directions, and wording of questions can be made.

Development, construction, and use of an educational game can be both a fun and profitable way to spend classroom time. Games can be produced for a wide variety of purposes and to meet the particular needs of students. If you haven't yet used this technique, why not give it a try?

Health 4 Fun: A Game of Knowledge

RAYMOND NAKAMURA teaches in the programs in physical education, School of Education, DePaul University, 1011 W. Belden Avenue, Chicago, Illinois 60614.

From time to time, as a diversion from standard methods, educational games can be excellent tools for learning. "Health 4 Fun" has been a successful game because it requires a lot of knowledge and provides some fun. It can be cooperative or competitive and can be used to develop research skills in dictionaries, encyclopedias, almanacs, textbooks, journals, etc.

The purpose of the game is to fill in the blanks of a play sheet with words or phrases that fit into pre-selected health categories. The filled-in words must begin with certain letters which are chosen at the beginning of the game.

The health categories chosen must suit the level of the class. Each one is written on a separate 3x5 index card. The cards are shuffled and placed face down; four cards are drawn from the pile. As each selection is read, all players write them down in the four category blanks on the play sheet.

Letters are written on another set of index cards, one per card. These are shuffled and four are drawn from the pile. The chosen letters are written in the appropriate blanks on the play sheet.

The Game

Each player tries to think of a word or phrase in each of the 16 blanks on the play sheet that fits the category at the top of the column and begins with the selected letters. An example of a filled-in play sheet follows. To add excitement, a time limit of 2–5 minutes can be put on the game.

The game can be played as a form of solitaire or by the whole class. Teams can be made for more competitive or cooperative games.

At the end of the game, players should research the answers they could not fill in. Discussions often develop when students come up with words or phrases that the others are not familiar with. Answers may be challenged; then they must be verified by research.

In competitive games the play sheets can be scored by adding up the number of correct answers in each column, horizontally and vertically for a maximum score of 32.

Here are some suggested health categories.

1. Body systems, organs, and glands
2. Bones or muscles
3. Fruits and vegetables
4. Meats, nuts or fish
5. Dairy products
6. Ice cream flavors
7. American foods
8. Foreign foods
9. Diets
10. Fitness: names of sports
11. Fresh and saltwater fish
12. Types of transportation
13. Types of fuel
14. Pollutants: cigarette names
15. Pollutants: automobile names
16. Environmental pollutants
17. Germs or bacteria
18. Medical laboratory apparatus
19. Human diseases
20. Communicable diseases
21. Non-communicable diseases
22. Drugs, medicine tradenames
23. Slang for drugs or medicines
24. Over the counter drugs
25. Pollutants: detergents
26. Wines
27. Beer
28. Soft drink tradenames
29. Hospital names
30. Health related journals
31. Health book titles
32. Health authors
33. Famous health people, past
34. Famous health people, present
35. Health organizations or societies
36. Health agencies, offices or departments
37. Health related professions
38. Environment: mountains
39. Environment: extinct animals or birds
40. Environment: endangered species
41. Environment: rivers and lakes
42. Environment: national parks
43. Bakery products
44. Famous restaurants
45. Kitchen utensils
46. Health related household items
47. Things commonly found in the medicine cabinet
48. Health related words over seven letters
49. Breakfast cereals
50. Famous physicians
51. Chemicals found in the body
52. Articles of clothing
53. Plant names
54. Flower names
55. Category of your choice

The degree of difficulty of these categories should be related to the academic level of the class. Many can be refined to offer greater difficulty. For example, a generalized category like prescription drugs can be limited to barbiturates. However, I have found it necessary to include some easy categories to ensure some success.

Category	Human Disease	Bones and Muscles	Auto Trade Names	Medical Apparatus	
D	Diphtheria	Deltoid	Dodge	Dilator	→ 4
W	Whooping Cough				→ 1
F	Fabry's Disease	Fibula	Ford	Forceps	→ 4
L	Leukemia		Lincoln	Lens	→ 3
	4	2	3	3	24 Total Score

(left side label: Pre-selected Letters)

School Health Bee

Bernard S. Krasnow is assistant principal and supervisor of health education at Arturo Toscanini Junior High School in Bronx, New York.

Health education took a dramatic turn last year at Toscanini Junior High School in Bronx, New York. Our school inaugurated its first annual health bee in order to stimulate greater participation and interest in health education and in current health topics.

The project was created out of a desire to change the traditional assembly program so that an atmosphere of excitement would pervade the audience. The health education department held a conference devoted to this idea and it was decided to promote a school-wide health knowledge quiz. This would culminate in a series of grade auditorium programs designed to duplicate the fun and excitement of television quiz programs.

The school's health instructor, Mr. Pluchik, was designated as the teacher-in-charge for the project. He constructed a health knowledge test from our own curriculum which was administered to all the students during their health or science periods. The students who scored highest on this initial survey test were invited to a class winners' run-off. Fifty-five class winners appeared for the run-off test which was held after school. Those with five highest scores in each grade were then designated as finalists and invited to participate in the auditorium quiz programs the following week. They were given extra resources in the form of textbooks, pamphlets, etc., to study from in preparation for the contest.

The auditorium program was modeled after a television panel quiz program. The industrial arts department constructed an electrical response board so that a contestant who knew the answer

was able to press a button to make a light flash in front of him. Mr. Pluchik served as moderator and asked the questions. Three other teachers acted as judges. The questions for the final quiz were selected from among those in the initial survey and the run-off examinations.

There was great anticipation on the part of the contestants and the student body. Publicity had been extensive through public address messages, posters, and class announcements so that most of the students were eagerly awaiting the program. The contests were well received by the audience and seldom has there been more audience enthusiasm. The excitement was, in fact, so great that many times the audience inadvertently shouted out the answer. (We did, in fact, throw the questions to the audience if they were not answered correctly by the contestants.) The scoring was conducted by awarding one point for each question answered correctly. Each contestant had his own personal scoreboard that reflected his current total. This kept the audience posted on the current scores.

Each auditorium program was concluded by awarding a trophy to the health quiz winner of each grade, and the finalists received honor certificates. The school photographer was there to take pictures of all the winners and we plan to display these for publicity purposes.

Our original idea in initiating this project was to focus on health education and current health topics. We are sure that this school-wide program did just that. We are, however, promoting follow-up activities so that our initial efforts are long-lasting. Some of these activities include: establishing a health information reference center in our school library, publicizing the health quiz in the community, establishing a health award for graduation, and promoting health topics to be taught as part of the curriculum in other subjects.

We are also hoping that we can motivate other schools in our district (District 9) to conduct their own Health Bee and, perhaps, even a city-wide contest. We think that it is time to stimulate nationwide excitement for health education. Who knows, a National Health Education Bee may someday stand right alongside our National Spelling Bee.

Not Merely Nostalgia

RALPH EDWARDS *is professor of health education and dean of administration and planning, Kingsborough Community College, City University of New York, Brooklyn, New York 11235.*

In moods of nostalgia, I am reminded of my elementary school days when we studied health heroes which, if memory serves me, were offered us in pamphlets published by Metropolitan Life Insurance Company. Tales of great exploits by leaders of science and health, including Madame Curie, Louis Pasteur, Florence Nightingale, and Walter Reed, set an example for a generation of youth for concern for human wellbeing and a search for truth, and cannot be minimized or ignored. Studying the life history of famous individuals is a desirable teaching tool and certainly well-known to our academic colleagues. The fact that a famous Hollywood star or an athlete uses a particular deodorant, travels on a particular airline or dresses in a particular garment is valuable where it counts heavily in this society—in the pocketbook. Health educators might seriously consider turning back the clock, for at least part of their instruction, to the Charles Atlas, Babe Zaharias era, to get the attitudinal value and maturation for us in education.

Some may have seen a recent news item concerning Richard M. Eakin, Professor of Zoology at Berkeley, Dr. Eakin, in order to make his subject alive and more interesting, has developed a technique of dressing up in the costume of famous lecturers in areas of zoology. Gregor Mendel, William Beaumont, Charles Darwin, William Harvey, Louis Pasteur are among "guests" that Eakin brings to his students. While teachers cannot be expected to be actors, certainly the impressions made by this instructor and the favorable response of the students suggests a new slant on an old approach to content and impact.

For some time I have introduced courses in health education with a historical perspective. Within these historical perspectives, individuals were sin-

gled out for their contribution to understanding health. Aesculapius and Hippocrates were the heroes of ancient Greece; Celsus and Galen of Greco-Rome; Rhazes, Avicenna, and Moses Maimonides of the Byzantine era; Paracelsus, Vesalius, Pare, Harvey, of the Renaissance; Lind, Hunter, Pinel, Rush, Bright, Braid were the 17th and 18th century heroes of the Enlightenment. The 19th century was full of individual efforts of Europeans as depicted by Claude Bernard, John Snow, Ludwig Ignaz Semmelweis, Rudolf Virchow, Florence Nightingale, Louis Pasteur, Joseph Lister, Richard Kraft-Ebbing, Robert Koch, Paul Ehrlich, Sigmund Freud, and Havelock Ellis. Americans are well placed in the health hall of fame of the 19th century by such luminaries as William Beaumont, Ephraim McDowell, James Marion Sims, William Morton, Clara Barton, William Osler, William Welch, Walter Reed, William Halsted, Simon Flexner, and Walter Cannon.

American contemporaries of the 20th century do not pale when we mention them in comparison to earlier heroes. Howard A. Rusk spent a lifetime treating the physically disabled and educating the public about the importance of rehabilitation; Will and Charles Mayo developed the model for cooperative group medical practice; Paul Dudley White, cardiologist, exercise proponent and physician to a president; Benjamin Spock, baby doctor, child care expert, social critic; Carl and William Menninger, advocates of psychiatric treat-

ment; Karl Landsteiner discoverer of four blood types; Jonas Salk and Albert Sabin, researchers and developers of polio vaccine; C. Walter Lillehi, Arthur DeBakey, Denton Cooley, pioneers in artificial heart devices; Linus Pauling, chemist of molecular structure and advocate of vitamin C; Rachel Carson, who in *Silent Spring* (1962) documented the effects on the environment of synthetic organic insecticides (DDT) and herbicides; John Rock and Gregory Pincus developed a synthetic fertility hormone; Rene Dubos, biochemist and advocate of antibiotic therapy; and, Hans Selye, endocrinologist and exponent of the "stress theory" of disease.

We can add to the list above the yearly Nobel Prize winners in chemistry, medicine, and biology. We do have a large assembly of heroic figures who have spent their professional lives working to keep man healthy and fit. Their accomplishments can be recognized as a teaching device and as a technique for valuable discussion. Their efforts demand applause even in an era which glorifies the anti-hero in fiction, movies, and television. Acknowledging the contribution of real heroes and placing them in a setting of everyday living is an important contribution to the student of health education and to the average citizen.

In bringing the heroes forward, it is not so much a question of what we can contribute to their memory, but rather what remembering them can contribute to us and our teaching.

Health in Concert

This article was submitted by the Senior Health Education Seminar, spring quarter 1976, Bowling Green State University. It was edited by CLAY WILLIAMS, assistant professor of health education, Bowling Green State University, Bowling Green, Ohio 43403 and JUDY SCHEER, assistant professor of health education, University of Toledo, Toledo, Ohio 43606.

What do "Puff the Magic Dragon," "Dead Babies," and "Junkfood Junkie" have in common? These and other such popular songs are a fantastic means of learning about current health issues. A "health concert" is a means of developing health concepts by capitalizing on a popular pastime of today's youth—music.

Music has much appeal for the young and old alike. It can have a calming effect as well as an energizing effect. The topic range is as diverse as the performers themselves. Some approach life with sincerity and heartache while others emphasize humor or entertainment. Listening to music of entertainers like John Denver can create a greater understanding of human emotions, actions, philosophies, and lifestyles. By bringing music into the classroom students and teachers have the tools to elaborate upon the relationship between music and health.

Songs can be used to introduce a unit or to maintain interest during the course of a unit. For example, by using a song like "Junkfood Junkie" as a part of a nutrition unit, a teacher could easily develop several followup activities relating to the theme of the song. This song touches on the social aspects of America's eating habits—the fast food craze, health foods, junk foods, vitamin supplements, and convenience foods.

Using this song to introduce a unit, challenge students to see how many nutrition concepts are in the lyrics. Their lists of concepts could then be used as guidelines to develop an overview of the unit. The song could also serve as a springboard for group activities or individual projects to develop the practical aspects of nutrition. Students may want to survey local fast food chains to obtain data enabling them to compare quantity and nutritional value for the consumer dollar. They could also research nutritional information about foods mentioned in the song. Others may want to construct low calorie meal plans which would provide essential nutrients while allowing occasional indulgence in junk foods without fear of weight gain.

Peter, Paul, and Mary's song "Puff the Magic Dragon," can be focused on marijuana, mental health, value clarification, and understanding one's self and relationship with others, creating an opportunity for lively discussion as students are challenged to search for the numerous interpretations that are provided in the lyrics. Interesting comparisons can be drawn when students are asked to interpret these lyrics both before and after appropriate health units. Students could also be encouraged to express their feelings and knowledge, individually or collectively, in song.

Another application would be to develop a mood chart based on the students' feelings after listening to the song. From this exposure, a discussion could be focused on using alternatives as a means of achieving highs. After such discussions, one could give the students a video camera and allow them to express visually and to share various opportunities for achieving natural highs.

Examples of additional health units and some songs that might be used in each category are as follows:

Drugs
"Mother's Little Helper" Rolling Stones
"The No No Song" Ringo Starr

"Momma Told Me Not to Come" Three Dog Night
"The Needle and the Damage Done" Neil Young
Personal and Social Relations
"At Seventeen" Janis Ian
"Looking for the Right One" Elvis Presley
"Everything I Own" David Gates
Death
"Patches" Clarence Carter
"Ode to Billy Jo"
"Run Johnny Run"

Alcoholism
"What Can A Family Say" America
"Social Disease" Elton John
"Another Try" America
Safety
"Convoy" W. C. McCoy
"Dead Man's Curve" Carpenters
Mental Health
"Sweet Surrender" John Denver
"Twisted" Joni Mitchell
"Leave Me Alone" Helen Reddy
"Brain Damage" Pink Floyd
Environment
"Where Will the Children Play" Cat Stevens
"Big Yellow Taxi" Joni Mitchell
Nutrition
"Junk Food Junkie" Larry Grace
"Savoy Truffle" Beatles
Venereal Disease
"You Left Me Sore" Todd Rungren
Contraception
"Unborn Child" Seals and Croft
"The Pill" Loretta Lynn
Sex Education
"All the Girls Love Alice" Elton John
"Sweet Painted Lady" Elton John
Aging
"When I'm Sixty Four" Beatles
"Old Folks" (from Jacques Brel is alive and well and living in Paris)
"Today is the First Day of the Rest of My Life" John Denver

Suggestions to help make your health concert an effective learning experience are:

1. Use quality audio equipment
2. Screen the songs before they are played to the class
3. Make copies of the lyrics for the students
4. Be open to a variety of interpretations
5. Be aware of misconceptions that may be conveyed in a song
6. Try to use current or well-known songs so the students can identify with them
7. Do not overuse the strategy

Tuning In To Health Education

WARREN L. McNAB is assistant professor of health education, Department of Health and Physical Education, University of Houston, 3801 Cullen Blvd., Houston, Texas 77004.

Music can be used effectively in health teaching because today it incorporates what is taking place in "real life" and stimulates moods in both young and old. Lyrics tell of death, love, life, human relationships, sorrow, happiness, and many other emotional experiences.

In health education these particular topics, as well as several others, are dealt with in the physical, mental/emotional, and social makeup of health. Interpreting music in conjunction with the health education discipline requires students to critically analyze and describe for themselves, based upon their own interpretation of the song and lyrics, what message or mood is being conveyed.

One way in which we used music in health education was to have students interpret a song sung by Melissa Manchester entitled "Midnight Blue." Before playing the record divide the class into groups of four or five and give each student a copy of the lyrics to the song. The groups read along and listen carefully to the lyrics and interpret what is said by applying the song to a specific situation.

The three situations are: (1) A friend is contemplating suicide and is on a ledge ready to jump—you are there trying to persuade this person to stop his/her attempt; (2) there has been a recent death in your immediate family; (3) you and your husband/wife are contemplating, or are on the verge of getting a divorce. Each group is given one of these situations. Based upon their particular situation each group is to relate and interpret what the song's lyrics mean and how it can be tied into the topic of mental health. The song is played and the groups are given ten minutes to decide what the lyrics mean in relation to their assigned topic and how each situation deals with mental/emotional health. These ideas are then shared in a class discussion.

The following lines from Melissa Manchester's song "Midnight Blue" and the students' interpretations serve as an

example of how we applied and interpreted the three situations to the song.

Line 1—*Whatever it is—it'll keep till the morning*
Suicide: Things right now seem unbearable, but perhaps we can iron out the problem tomorrow. Give it one more chance.
Death: If we can just get through today's sadness and grief, tomorrow will be better.

Divorce: Can't our differences be settled tomorrow? Let's sleep on it and we may change our minds.

Line 2—*Haven't we both got better things to do?*
Suicide: You have a purpose in life, you can be somebody, you will hurt others by what you are doing; there is much more in life to experience.
Death: One must go on in life; death is part of living.
Divorce: Can't we try something else besides divorce?

Line 3—*Midnight blue*
Suicide:
Death: Dark, black, fearful, mysterious
Divorce: time of one's life

Line 4—*Even the simple things become rough*
Suicide: Everyone has problems in life. At any one time we may think life is not worth living, but we can adjust to most problems. Suicide won't resolve these problems.
Death: Even though we know death is coming, it is extremely difficult to accept.
Divorce: Every little thing hurts at times like this; there is no simple solution.

This approach to teaching allows students to interpret the message stated in the song and through individual and collective thinking apply their interpretation and feelings to a health related situation. "Midnight Blue" is effective in looking at the different, and yet similar, mental/

emotional problems that are dealt with in a crisis such as suicide, death, or divorce. Followup questions which are brought up can be directly tied into their discussions, for example: How do you *feel* after listening to the song? How do emotions affect one's life? How can emotions be beneficial in one situation and destructive in another? Can music relieve or create stress and tension? What emotions are elicited from you by this song in relation to suicide, death, divorce? How do emotions affect one's behavior? How does one's mental/emotional health affect one's physical and social health?

These are basic questions that are dealt with in the topic of mental health, but the use of music allows students to relate to this information and apply it in a relevant manner. In addition, environmental influences of one's mental health, and how music does indeed affect one's emotional health in both positive and negative aspects of life can be discussed.

Other song possibilities and their related topics are "When I'm Sixty Four" (by John Lennon and Paul McCartney) for aging, "Lighting Bar Blues" (by Arlo Guthrie) for alcohol use, "I Love You" (by Olivia Newton John) for human relationships, "Poems, Prayers and Promises" (by John Denver) for mental health, and "Junkfood Junkie" (by Larry Grace) for nutrition.

Students can also be asked to bring in a record which they feel has a health message or could be applied to a health topic. This particular method of teaching allows for individual thinking, a sharing of ideas, and it stimulates students making health education a fun, relevant and worthwhile experience.

Ideas for Successful Health Teaching*

LOREN B. BENSLEY, JR. is associate professor of health education, Central Michigan University, Mt. Pleasant, Michigan 48858.

As a professor of teaching methods, I am a great believer that how you teach is just as important as what you teach. Many times, we teach the way we were taught, rather than the way we were taught to teach. In order for health teaching to be successful, it is of utmost importance that the methods used be creative and original in every possible way. By doing this, the subject will be more interesting to the students and enhance the opportunities for behavior change. It is important that the material presented to the students be student centered rather than subject centered.

In the past ten years of teaching health education to secondary school and university students, I have discovered four essential points for successful health teaching. First, learning must be enjoyable. If the students find that learning health can be fun, it is then correct to assume that they will enter into the learning experience with a great deal of enthusiasm and excitement. Second, students must become emotionally involved in the learning process. This can be done rather easily in teaching health education; one's health is a personal thing and to become involved emotionally in the subject matter is almost automatic. The third point to consider in teaching health education is that the student should be granted a degree of academic freedom to explore his or her own health needs and interests. By so doing, the student experiences health learning as something which becomes relevant and has a purpose.

*The information in this article is based on material which appeared originally in a column entitled "Ideas for Successful Health Teaching" published in the *Journal* of the Michigan Association for Health, Physical Education, and Recreation. The *MAHPER Journal* editor, Joan Nelson, granted permission for its use.

For this to happen, it is necessary for the teacher to create an atmosphere of freedom without external threats. The fourth essential point in teaching health education is the need for the teacher to know his students. This point cannot be stressed enough. In order for a health teacher to experience success to any degree, it is necessary that he design the course with a full understanding of the students' health needs and interests. The health educator must gather data on the personal health habits, attitudes, and behaviors of those students he is teaching at any one time.

These four points are only a part of successful health teaching; they are mentioned here because oftentimes teachers overlook what might be considered the obvious items in teaching. With these points in mind, it is interesting to explore some different ways to teach health education to secondary school students, such as the following two methods I have found to be successful.

Using Popular Music In Teaching Health

Much of today's popular music has a great deal of meaning behind the strange sounds and muddled voices. By examining some of the music subscribed to by today's youth, the teacher will discover that much is written about drug abuse, human sexuality, environmental conditions, and mental and emotional health. It is suggested that the teacher listen to some of the songs from the very popular and successful rock musical "Hair." The song "Pollution" is concerned with air pollution, whereas the song "Sodomy" refers to human sexuality. This topic is also discussed in the lyrics of music composed by current popular artists such as Mick Jagger and the Rolling Stones, in "Live With Me" or "Let's Spend the Night Together." The group called The Rare Earth also sings about sexuality in their song titled "In Bed." Music about sexuality is extensive, and the health educator can be selective in choosing songs pertaining

to homosexuality, sexual intercourse, or fellatio.

Within the last few years the song "I Never Promised You a Rose Garden" became very popular. This song could be played in class and discussed in relation to mental and emotional health. The discussion could center around the fact that no one promises you everything and you must work for much that you receive in life. For a unit on mental health the author has experienced success with a ninth grade health education class using some of Simon and Garfunkel's work, notably, the songs "Bridge Over Troubled Water," "A Most Peculiar Man," and "Richard Cory." The latter two are pertinent to the topic of suicide. The students' favorite song pertaining to mental health, however, is "Walk a Mile in My Shoes" by Joe South.

The teacher can also talk about musicians or musical groups and center the discussion around the use of drugs. For example, several years ago two very popular musicians died of an overdose of drugs. The class might discuss the questions why Janis Joplin and Jimmy Hendrix used drugs and eventually took an overdose.

The use of popular music as a medium to teach health has been extremely interesting to me and my students. One reason is because the teacher is using a significant object of the teenagers' life—his music. It is, in effect, a way of reaching students through their own medium.

Using Current and Popular Literature in Teaching Health

Just as effective as using popular music in teaching health education is the use of popular literature. Are there any books you have read in the past year which could be used to teach about health? Often there is a novel, fictional story, biography, or some piece of literature that contains information pertinent to a health education class. When discussing drug abuse, students may read the book *Valley of the Dolls*, a story about barbiturate addiction and the eventual death of the main character of the story. When discussing the topic of love and personal relationships, the ever popular novel *Love Story* is suggested to the students. This particular story, about two young people who fall in love and marry, is good because of the deep, meaningful feeling the couple have toward each other. It is essential when discussing emotions in regard to human sexuality that mature love be understood. The book *Love Story* brings this out.

There are hundreds of books that could be used for discussion purposes in a health education course. The important things when considering this method are first, that the teacher select a book which is suitable to the subject at hand and, second, that it has appeal to the students. It is both a real challenge and an enjoyable way of teaching.

The Student Interview Technique

MARC E. MEYER is a health education teacher at North Rockland High School, Hammond Road, Thiells, New York 10984.

As health educators we are always looking for ways to encourage class participation. One method seems to work quite well within my health education classes—the "student interview technique."

This technique works well because it has certain qualities which help students in a variety of ways. First, the technique is flexible, each teacher can use the interview for a particular unit or simply for a change of pace in daily routines. Second, it allows each student to communicate his/her ideas to others. It helps develop

dents and the individuals who conducted the interview will tell what they discovered.

I have found that there are a variety of ways one can use this technique. Each teacher should choose that method which best suits his/her situation. The interview can be specific, (drugs, alcohol, sex education, mental health) or general, asking questions as presented here, which explore a variety of ideas and values.

By implementing activities such as the "student interview technique," students come away from class with a better feeling; most were eager to participate and most had a positive learning experience which they will not soon forget.

Interview #1

Instructions:

Interview two individuals in your class. You are not to give more than two interviews.

Interview #2

Instructions:

Interview two individuals in your class. You are not to give more than two interviews.

Questions:

Name?
What three things do you prize most?
If you could visit anywhere in the world, where would it be?
If you could divide $5,000 between two charities, what would they be?
When was the last time you were punished?
Why were you punished?
Do you have many friends?
What do you feel was the best movie you ever saw?
What is important to you?
When was the last time you gave advice to someone?
Did he/she ask for your advice?

the ability to communicate and to listen, as well as to stimulate class discussion.

In speaking with my students, a number of them have said that they find the student interview, "interesting," "makes time go faster," "gives us a chance to learn more about our friends," and it is "fun." Of the many activities and options available to my classes, the "student interview technique" allows for a great range of communication and interaction within the classroom.

Below are examples of interviews used at different times throughout the semester. The interview sheet clearly tells each student to interview two individuals within the class. No student is to give more than two interviews. Upon completion, the teacher can simply call on stu-

Questions:

Name?
What was the happiest time of your life?
What do you like to do with your free time?
Favorite musical group?
Things you like best about being in high school?
Brothers and sisters (how many)?
Where do you like to go with your friends?
What is your favorite food?
If you had a million dollars, how would you spend it?
What is your favorite sport?

Interview #3

Instructions:

Interview two individuals in your class. You are not to give more than two interviews.

Questions:

Name?
What time do you get up each day?
What time do you go to sleep?
Favorite TV program?
When was the last time you gave someone a compliment?
Is it difficult to give compliments?
Is "time" important to you?
What was the most frightening movie you ever saw?
Which was the saddest movie you ever saw?
Are you on time for appointments?

Positive Peer Influence: School-Based Prevention

AIDA K. DAVIS is a research assistant and JOAN M. WEENER is a project assistant in the Addictions Prevention Laboratory and ROBERT E. SHUTE is assistant professor of health education. They are all at Pennsylvania State University, University Park, Pennsylvania 16802.

Peer pressure is often considered a psychological force—a direct attempt by a group to influence personal behaviors of group members. However, Kiesler and Kiesler[1] have a somewhat broader view which acknowledges unplanned, but nevertheless, highly controlling influences of groups: "All that is required is that the group expect the person to act or believe in a certain way, or that the person think such things are expected of him."

Whether peer influence is defined as psychological forces or group sanctions, the mechanisms and effects are inextricably bound to the operations of social influence, which include teaching, learning, imparting ideas and skills, generating enthusiasm and purpose, and even the application of force. Peer influence and the conformity it engenders is part of a much larger context of cognitive and motivational processes related to social learning.

While any social interaction is potentially influential the greatest power to dispense social rewards and punishments to the individual member is attributed to peer group interactions. It is within the peer group that the effects of social modeling and behavioral shaping tend to be most concentrated. Especially for adolescent and college-aged people, the peer group is often cited as the primary reference group for attitudes, values, and behaviors; it is within the peer group that outside influences (parents, the law, the schools, etc.) are discussed, judged, and mediated. Acquiescence to direct or subtle pressures in peer groups has been linked to some forms of juvenile delinquency, truancy, malicious mischief, sexual experimentation, drug use, and other types of misbehavior directed against self or society.

While the motivation for initiation and continuation of drug use and the conditions under which drug attitudes and behaviors are learned are as varied as the social, religious, educational, occupational, and psychological backgrounds of the user, many writers are now emphasizing the critical role of peer influence as a variable which may override many of these considerations.[2]

Researchers in high schools and colleges have found that the likelihood of personal drug use correlates highly with the drug-using activities of one's peer group. This fact has influenced the development of a variety of school-based peer programs related to student performance and student attitude toward teachers, school, self, and others. The underlying assumption is that if students have a healthy self-concept, a favorable attitude toward their teacher and schools, a number of satisfying and enhancing interpersonal relationships with family and friends, and are comfortable about their values and abilities to make decisions, then they are much less likely to succumb to pressures which encourage self-destructive behaviors.

Several school-based programs have evolved which draw on some of the positive aspects of peer influence. For example, peer and cross-age tutoring and peer counseling, while not specifically oriented toward prevention of drug and alcohol abuse, seek to reduce behavioral problems and bridge the gap between student and teacher (or parents) by providing individualized instruction, personal interactions, and counseling. The school can include exercises which help students discuss and understand the "mechanisms" of peer influence and help them develop skills to deal with influential situations. All of these programs or strategies are meant to develop the individual's sense of personal competence and responsibility. Following are several workable strategies and resources for involving peers in prevention activities in the school setting.

Peer/Cross-age Tutoring

Peer and cross-age tutoring has been included in school programs for a long time as a way of meeting special educational needs. Historically pupils helped or taught other children in order to alleviate the responsibilities and time constraints of the teacher in the one-room schoolhouse. Later, the idea of students helping each other proved to be a promising alternative in traditional schools. The trained tutor was able to establish a personal relationship with other students and could assist them with their school work for both remedial and standard purposes. The learner was able to receive help in a variety of academic areas, while the tutors found that the teaching provided a powerful learning experience for themselves as well.

Tutoring programs vary widely in relationship to the age differences which exist between tutor and pupil. "Peer tutoring" connotes that tutors are the same age or are enrolled in the same course as the learners, whereas older students or students who had completed the course or were not enrolled in it at the same time as the pupils were defined as "cross-tutors."[3]

Tutoring techniques have been promoted as a means of enhancing the learning of both tutor and learner, though some researchers have urged caution in making this claim.[4] Tutoring responsibilities and establishing a close personal relationship with the learner are important affective gains for the student tutor. Opportunities for creating constructive, social, and positive roles, greatly enhance the tutor's school experience.[5] The learner's gains in academic skills and understanding seem to promote self-esteem.

Tutoring as a preventive approach to drug and alcohol abuse relies on the concomitant development of skills which ultimately enhance the student's personal satisfaction with life. These skills include *intra*personal aspects such as improved self-concept, as well as *inter*personal skills—effective communication with others, sharing personal difficulties, etc.

Resources. Many aspects involved in designing and implementing a tutoring program are discussed in a variety of training guides available to schools. The

National Commission on Resources for Youth under the direction of Mary Kohler has developed a tutoring project called "Youth Tutoring Youth." Several hundred programs have been started in schools and by community agencies across the nation. Over 3,500 persons have been trained in the techniques of tutoring through this flexible program which can be adjusted to meet the needs of school or community groups.[6]

The Ontario-Montclair School District in California has developed a cross-age teaching manual designed to help teachers or administrators organize and implement a tutoring program. This manual describes agendas for training seminars and the matching procedure for older and younger students as well as describing scheduling, types of activities, and cost considerations.[7]

A further guide to tutoring is included in volume two of *Balancing Head and Heart: Sensible Ideas for the Prevention of Drug and Alcohol Abuse.*[8] These books were produced for Pennsylvania's Governor's Council on Drug and Alcohol Abuse and contain a general rationale for primary prevention along with descriptions of eleven school-based approaches to prevention of drug abuse, including peer tutoring and peer counseling. Sensible guidelines for implementing strategies and providing resources make this publication a handy reference guide.

Peer Counseling

Another activity, defined by M. G. Sussman, which capitalizes on the positive effects of peer influence, is peer counseling: "a process in which trained and supervised students offer listening, support, and alternatives and other verbal and non-verbal interaction, but little or no advice, to students who refer themselves."[9] Peer counseling programs are usually designed as supportive programs which complement or supplement existing guidance programs in the schools. While including academics, peer counseling programs are generally aimed at clarification of feelings, ideas, and values in order to enhance personal decision-making and resolution. Trained students provide a climate of acceptance for those fellow students who would rather share problems with a peer than with an adult.

Junior and senior high school students are trained in reflective listening skills, problem solving, and providing information or referral if needed, by school counselors, teachers, or psychologists. Training methods consist primarily of supervised seminars or workshops for selected student volunteers. In some schools the training courses are given for credit, others provide training on an extracurricular basis. A number of programs have established a general "rap room," "drop-in center" or "unwinding room" where students are welcome to come and talk about their concerns. Appointments can also be made for private sessions with one of the peer counselors. This type of program expands available counseling resources and makes it easier for students to discuss problems on a less formal basis. Counselors are trained to recognize and refer students with serious problems to professional counselors.

Resources. A variety of training materials are available for help in implementing peer counseling programs. Samuels and Samuels' book is a thorough review of rationale, needs, organization, and evaluation of peer counseling.[10] The authors provide a detailed account for interested administrators and participants. The *Balancing Head and Heart* series notes the benefits for both counselors and counselees in communication skills, self-confidence, and self-esteem.

Newsletters such as the one distributed by the National Resources for Youth[11] cover a number of projects in which teenagers counsel their peers. A prevention resource bulletin, "Pyramid," sponsored by the Prevention Branch of the National Institute on Drug Abuse reviews and reports on peer tutoring and counseling prevention programs.[12] A manual entitled *Teen Involvement: A Teen Counselor Training Manual* by Gladys Conroy contains a number of ideas for training teen counselors to work in the area of drug and alcohol abuse prevention.[13]

Integrated Classroom Experiences

More informal, planned interventions in the classrooms, which integrate normal lessons with opportunities for student growth in dealing with situations involving peer and/or social influence, offer attractive, inexpensive starting points for peer prevention programming.

Photo: NEA Communication Services

47

Peer Influence   "Convince Me"   Time: 35 minutes

Purpose: To have students develop an awareness of how they influence and are influenced by their peers.

Materials: One mimeographed sheet for each student in the class. Half of the sheets should have the following written on them:

Role A—You've just left a home basketball game. Your older sister, who's obviously drunk, pulls over and says she wants to show you and your friend how fast her new car can go on a back road near town. You love the feel of speeding and are anxious to accept her offer, so although you think your friend is probably chicken, you try to convince him/her that he/she would be a fool not to go along.

The other half of the sheets should have this written on them:

Role B—You're a fairly shy person and don't want to have anything to do with what your friend suggests.

Procedure
1. Pass Role A out to half the class, Role B to the other half of the class, asking students to keep their role secret.
2. Have each student with a Role A sheet pair up with a student with a Role B sheet. If there is an uneven number, have the extra student watch two others role play.
3. Give students about five minutes to play their roles.
4. Now have students trade roles and again spend about five minutes playing the opposite role.
5. Ask students to return to their seats and have a class discussion about how they felt in each role.
6. Discussion hints:
a. How did you feel in each role?
b. What did your partner do to make you feel that way?
c. What are some pros and cons of trying to get others to do things we want them to do?
d. Under what circumstances would you try to convince a friend to do something?
e. What do you gain when you give in? What do you lose?

Adaptations:
1. Add more roles so that two or three students can try to convince classmates to do something they do not want to do. Have the students rotate roles within the group.
2. Have three students try to convince three other students to do something they do not want to do. The activities can be modified e.g., taking drugs; going swimming in fast, cold water; exploring a cave, etc.

Integration Suggestions: Role playing is so versatile and enjoyable that you should find students eager to participate and initiate suggestions. A few possibilities are:

1. Mathematics—Devise roles for students so they may try to convince others of the "best" way to invest $10,000. The setting could be a board of directors meeting for a small business.
2. Art—Devise roles for the artist, the merchant, the buyer, and the skeptic. Have the artist try to convince the merchant to display his creation. Have the merchant try to convince the buyer to buy it. Have the buyer try to convince a skeptical friend that he/she has made a wise purchase. A funny painting or sculpture would be an asset to the exercise. Discuss the motivation of each person in the role-play scene.

Contributed by Liz Kramer and Robert Shute

During the past year, a review of the research and existing curricular resources which relate directly to aspects of peer pressure/peer influence was conducted as a task of the Peer Pressure Project (funded by the Addictions Prevention Laboratory and directed by Robert E. Shute). The project staff will have adapted a number of flexible lesson plans from existing resources or will have created new ones when the project is completed.[14] These lesson plans will form one section of a teacher resource package for integrating peer influence lessons into a classroom. A sample lesson with integration suggestions is presented here.

We know of no other compilation of strategies similar to the one being developed for the Peer Pressure Project. Certainly, many excellent ideas for integrating peer influence study can be found in recent texts, curriculum guides, and audiovisual materials on related topics—affective education, humanistic education, developmental education, and confluent education. Several peer-related exercises can be adapted from the wealth of existing materials which schools can use to enhance learning, improve decision-making skills, clarify values, etc., at all educational levels. Generally, these have come to be highly regarded as valid enhancers of the educational experience.

Alternative Peer-Related Activities

A number of other peer-related activities such as drop-in centers, alternatives-for-youth programs, vocational skills training, and youth service programs have been developed in both school and community settings. These programs encourage activities which provide meaningful alternatives to drug and alcohol use. Program goals may range from developing clearly defined skills, such as photography, macrame or dancing, to experiencing and sharing insight and ideas with peers and becoming involved in service to others. The concept of service to others as a developmental goal for schools has been acknowledged by Kohler:

> Our schools are no longer filling the needs of our children. A generation ago, living itself provided opportunities for youngsters to be with adults, to grasp the satisfaction of work. Today we stick kids in a world of their own and tell them to stay where they are until we need them. Despite the increased number of "people needs" in our complex society, adolescents aren't given a chance to "help out." We must link the teen-agers into the system—and give them opportunities to help meet human needs.[15]

Alternative projects for peers, along with peer tutoring, peer counseling, and classroom activities, draw strength as prevention activities by using positive peer models rather than focusing on a specific social and/or health related problem.

Resources. For those who wish to become more familiar with alternative peer and prevention approaches the following publications are recommended. *Alternative Pursuits for America's 3rd Century: A Resource Book on Alternatives to Drugs* provides a guide to possible projects. The section entitled "Alternatives" in the *Balancing Head and Heart* series offers ideas for teenage projects. *Youth Alternatives*, the monthly newsletter of the National Youth Alternatives Project, offers descriptions of programs as well as funding opportunities and legislative action reports.[16]

The encouraging research and program evaluations point toward the efficiency of using peers as change agents for the prevention of drug and alcohol abuse. Likewise, the translation of the "positive peer influence" concept to other health related or social problems such as contraception behavior, smoking, reckless driving, etc., should be seriously considered when planning school or community prevention programs.

[1]Kiesler, C. and Kiesler, S. *Conformity.* Reading, Mass.: Addison Wesley Publ., 1969.

[2]Dumont, M. "Mainlining America: Why the Young Use Drugs." *Social Policy*, November/December 1971, pp. 36–40.

[3]Deterline, W. A. *Training and Management of Student Tutors*. ERIC Document Reproduction Service, No. ED 048 133, 1970.

[4]Willis, J. and Crowder, J. "Does Tutoring Enhance the Tutor's Academic Learning?" *Psychology in the Schools*, 1974, II(1), pp. 68–70.

[5]Gartner, A.; Kohler, M. C.; and Riessman, F. "Every Child a Teacher," *Childhood Education*, 1971, pp. 12–16.

[6]*Youth Tutoring Youth: A Manual for Trainers*. National Commission on Resources for Youth, 36 West 44th St., New York, 1970.

[7]*A Cross-age Teaching Resource Manual*, Ontario-Montclair School District, 950 West D St., Ontario, Calif., 1971.

[8]*Balancing Head and Heart: Sensible Ideas for the Prevention of Drug and Alcohol Abuse*, Pacific Institute for Research and Evaluation, Suite 201, Quail Ct., Walnut Creek, Calif., 1975.

[9]Samuels, J. and Samuels, D. *The Complete Handbook of Peer Counseling*, Miami, Fla.: Fiesta Publ., 1975, p. 41.

[10]*Ibid*.

[11]*Resources for Youth*, National Commission on Resources for Youth, 36 West 44th St., New York.

[12]*Pyramid*, Pacific Institute for Research and Evaluation, Walnut Creek, Calif.

[13]Conroy, G. *Teen Involvement: A Teen Counselor Training Manual*. New York: Holt, Rinehart and Winston, 1972.

[14]Shute, R. E. *Explorations in Social and Peer Influence: A Resource Manual for Teachers—Grades 7–10*, 1977.

[15]*Alternative Pursuits for America's 3rd Century: A Resource Book on Alternatives To Drugs*, National Institute on Drug Abuse, Washington, D.C., 1974, p. 2.

[16]*Youth Alternatives*, National Youth Alternatives Project, Inc., 1346 Connecticut Ave., NW, Washington, D.C.

Ernie

LILLIAN D. FESPERMAN is a graduate assistant in health and physical education, Miami University, Oxford, Ohio 45056.

Are you tired of teaching digestion, respiration, circulation, the body systems and functions the same way year after year, class after class? Or are you an inexperienced teacher looking for a new approach for old, unchanging yet vital material? In either case, here is a successful, exciting, beneficial solution which can motivate your students.

When I was teaching health at Alexander Graham Junior High School in Charlotte, North Carolina, I was a first year teacher willing to try just about anything that would motivate my students. I had to present a unit on the systems of the body and wanted to try a new, creative approach. After evaluating possibilities, I came up with the idea of constructing a body in class.

Selling my idea to the students was extremely easy and well-received; everyone wanted to "build a body." We first got basic background information on the systems of the body and gathered our ideas and materials for building a body. We included five systems—digestive, skeletal, respiratory, circulatory, and nervous—on our body. Since there were five seventh grade health classes, each class contributed one system to the body.

Information about systems was covered in class by a series of handouts, lectures, discussions, pictures, and films. Students were required to keep a notebook related to the systems which they handed in at the end of the unit. To further instill interest in the students, as we discussed the systems I mentioned ideas and suggestions about the body that we could try. We all knew we were working to gather enough information to construct a life-size body out of a variety of "raw" materials.

After completing the general background information, a system was assigned to each class and that class was responsible for bringing in any materials related to their system. They were also required to read books and study pictures and charts related to their systems. Specific tasks were assigned to small groups, who worked together to make their particular system fit into the body.

The skeletal system included the pelvic bone, upper and lower bones of the arms, finger bones, upper and lower leg bones, the kneecap, the sternum, collarbone, and back vertebrae. The nervous system had the brain and spinal cord, and nerves. Our digestive system was made up of the tongue and esophagus, spleen, liver, stomach, small intestine, large intestine, and the rectum. The nasal cavity, trachea, bronchial tubes, and lungs (one open and one closed) with alveoli were the

"Ernie", created by seventh grade students.

parts of the respiratory system. The circulatory system consisted of the heart, aorta, large and small veins, and arteries.

We needed a base on which to mount our body parts. After considering the possibilities of cardboard, wood and other hard material, we decided to use a big sheet of plywood so we could attach the organs and have them stay in place. The plywood (about 5' by 3') was supplied by one student's parents. We cut out a body frame from paper, glued it onto the plywood and started assembling organs and parts.

The materials brought in by the classes for use included chicken bones, styrofoam of all sizes and shapes, sponges, thread of assorted colors, wire and plastic-coated wires of various colors and sizes, clay, newspaper, paints, cardboard cylinders, empty thread

spools, balloons, nails, cloth scrap, glue, and toothpicks.

We made some of our bones out of sticks covered with papier maché, and others with styrofoam cut into the shapes of the bones we wanted. The bones were attached to the body frame first along with the trachea, which we made from a cardboard cylinder wrapped in yarn for the cartilage, and the bronchial tubes, which were made from clay. The digestive system was then attached. The tongue was a small, semi-inflated balloon; the esophagus was a small cardboard tube fitted inside the trachea. The stomach and large intestines were papier maché wrapped over blown up balloons. The balloons were then deflated and the papier maché organs cut in half to make a flat surface to mount on the plywood body. The small intestine, liver, and spleen were made out of clay which was dried and painted, then nailed or glued onto the frame. The nasal cavity was cardboard cut into shape, the bronchial tubes were clay, and the lungs were styrofoam. One lung was painted as if it were closed, the other lung was constructed as if it were open. The capillaries were drawn with magic marker and little pieces of sponge glued on it to show the alveoli.

The heart was made by cutting the shape out of a thick sponge, with veins and arteries drawn into it. The pulmonary vein and artery and the aorta were inserted into the sponge with big red and blue wires. From the heart came red and blue arteries and veins made from wire and thread. Veins and arteries not made of wire or thread were drawn on the body with red and blue pens. The nervous system was done with various colored wires for the nerves leading all through the body to the fingers and feet. The spinal cord was made of yellow yarn leading from the brain, which was a piece of plastic cauliflower since the bumps and shape were similar. We cut the cauliflower to make a flat back surface to fit onto the frame. It was definitely an authentic-looking part of the body.

All of the parts were either glued, taped, or nailed into place on the body frame. The bones were mounted first with the trachea, esophagus, and bronchial tubes. Then the lungs, heart, and digestive system was fitted into place. The veins, arteries, and nerves were intertwined into place last, making our body complete. The classes then named our project body "Ernie."

Other suggestions for materials that we did not include in our project that could be added to yours are a mop for hair, or maybe garden hose for intestines. Or how about bottle caps or ping-pong balls for eyes? Other ideas may be to use false teeth or plastic ears to make your body more complete.

The project was stimulating and interesting to the students. The students responsible for making system parts and placing them onto the body also had to explain the operations of the organ or part. They benefited greatly from this project by learning about the human body and working together and had fun doing it. It is an excellent idea to try in your own classroom. Why not create your own "Ernie"?

Focus on Content

Empathizing With Addicts

PETER FINN is senior education and training analyst at ABT Associates, Inc., 55 Wheeler Street, Cambridge, Massachusetts 02138.

Most people who have never experienced a major addiction such as, alcoholism, drug dependence, compulsive eating, or cigarette smoking, have little understanding and often many misconceptions about what it feels like to have a persistent and irresistible craving for a substance or activity. An addiction is defined here as a craving for a substance or activity which a person cannot at the moment resist consistently or for a sustained period of time. In the following learning exercise, students gain insight into the nature of addictions by refraining for an agreed-upon period of time from an activity they have found extremely enjoyable for some time. As a result of this period of "abstinence," students may be better able to appreciate what an addicted person feels like and how they can best help relatives and friends who may have a dependency.

The exercise may also enable some students to realize that they have a strong and perhaps ungovernable urge for a substance or activity and to consider whether their compulsive behavior is healthy and what causes it. The exercise can foster insight into why everyone feels dependent on some activities and provide an inkling of how the students may feel if they are some day deprived of a substance or activity to which they have become accustomed or addicted.

This exercise has been used many times by me at the junior and senior high school level. However, it probably would be successful with elementary school students and adult groups, as well.

Procedure

Have students pick one or two activities which they would find very difficult—perhaps impossible—to stop doing. Then have each student agree in a written contract with the rest of the class to forego the activity for at least a week, but preferably for a month. It might be more enjoyable and educational for students to experiment with a friend or small group, with each person renouncing the same activity. Depending on their "passions," students might:

use no salt or sugar in their food

give up cigarettes

stop seeing or talking with a close friend

not kiss or touch their girlfriend, boyfriend, husband, or wife

not make or answer any telephone calls

get up at 4:00 a.m. every morning (not sleep late)

stop watching television or listening to the radio

give up Coke, coffee, or another favorite beverage

give up a favorite sport or other form of recreation

stop chewing gum

It may be helpful for the students to keep a diary of their behavior and feelings during the experiment to jog their memory when they relate their experiences to the class. Students can also talk into a tape recorder at the end of each day and play back excerpts to the class at the conclusion of the experiment.

Follow-up Discussion

After students have refrained from their activities for at least a week, have the class recount their experiences, then answer the following questions.

1. How many of you succeeded in refraining from your activities for the entire period of time stipulated in your contracts? How soon did those who failed give in? How do those of you who failed give in? How do those of you who failed feel about yourselves—disappointed? angry? indifferent? relieved? How do those of you who succeed feel—superior? sympathetic? resentful? neutral?

2. What did not doing the activity feel like? Did you miss it badly? Did you get angry? frightened? miserable? grouchy? bored? frustrated?

3. Did your relationships with other people change? For example, did you avoid certain people, or people in general, spend more time than usual with certain people, or with people in general, or relate to people differently such as, arguing more than normally?

4. Did talking or being with other students who were refraining from the same activity (or a different activity) help you resist the temptation to give in? Did you ask for, and get, help from other people in your attempts to forego the activity? How did they respond? How would you have liked them to respond?

5. Did other people change their behavior, attitudes, or feelings toward you as a result of your experiment? How did you feel about and react to that?

6. Did you start doing things that you don't usually do, such as forget things, become less observant, overeat, or develop physical symptoms such as headaches, stomach aches, tics, loss of appetite, insomnia, or unusual fatigue?

7. Did your other activities change at all? Did you compensate for the lack of your "forbidden" activity by participating more in some other pursuit? Did the substitute activity help take your mind off the thing you wanted to do? Did your efforts at compensation affect any of the people around you?

8. Were you confronted with an opportunity to "lapse," and did your willpower diminish in the presence of the forbidden activity or object? Were other people considerate in not mentioning the activity or substance, or helpful in suggesting a substitute?

9. Did you go out of your way to avoid the activity or substance, or things that might remind you of it? Did your avoidance behavior help reduce your craving?

10. Did you cheat at all? If so, did you try to engage in your activity just a little and find you couldn't resist resuming it completely? Did you bother to hide your lapses from other people? If so, did anyone catch you cheating? How did they react? How did you feel about being discovered?

11. When you finally did go back to the activity, how did it feel? Did you try to "make up for lost time"?

After the class has explored the issues related to these questions, students can discuss how their actions and feelings might be similar to those of an alcoholic, drug addict, cigarette smoker, compulsive eater, or other addicted person. The group should also consider how its experiences may have been different from those of truly addicted people. For example, the students knew they could resume their activity with impunity at the end of the test period, while an alcoholic, who has stopped drinking or an obese person who has begun dieting knows that to revert to their former behavior is to court disaster.

Students may also erroneously conclude, based on their own success, that addicted people should be able with relative ease to reject their self-destructive practices. The students' experience may have misled them because their own craving was a comparatively mild one and made even more bearable by the realization that it was only temporary.

Finally, focus specifically on how the students feel about addicted people. Do they feel the same way about alcoholics or drug addicts as they felt about themselves during their experiment? Should they? Did they gain any new insights into what it feels like to have an addiction and how addicted people can best be helped to shake off their dependency? Were the students able to identify any compulsive behaviors of their own and gain a better understanding of how to evaluate and cope with them?

How Much Can I Drink?

H. RICHARD TRAVIS is assistant professor of health science, James Madison University, Harrisonburg, Virginia 22802.

I teach drug education courses and frequently, when discussing alcohol, students will ask how much a person can drink before being considered drunk. I point out that there are many variables that influence the extent to which an individual will be affected by alcohol.

1. Some people are affected more than others because of their biochemical make-up.

2. The attitude or mood of the individual at the time of drinking as well as the environment in which alcohol is drunk influence the effect.

3. Food and liquid in the stomach dilute the alcohol and slow down its absorption.

4. The carbon dioxide in carbonated alcoholic beverages tends to hasten the movement of the alcohol from the stomach through the pylorus to the small intestine where the majority of alcohol is absorbed.

5. The blood alcohol level reached in the body is related to the individual's body weight. A larger person has more body fluids and blood to dilute alcohol than a smaller person. The more alcohol in the blood, the more that can diffuse into the cells of the body. Most states set 0.1% as the blood alcohol level at which a person is considered legally drunk.

A number of charts are available in textbooks or from state divisions of motor vehicles which relate the number of drinks a person consumes to weight and subsequent blood alcohol level. I use the following chart to have students calculate what their blood alcohol level might be after a certain number of drinks and the number of minutes since they first started drinking. Most students know their body weight, but if not, a scale can be brought into the room for them. They follow these steps to figure their blood alcohol level.

1. Emphasize that this chart is a guide and not a guarantee. Remind the class of the variables that have been listed.

2. If your weight is between two of those shown on the chart, use the lower weight.

3. On the chart, look up the blood alcohol level associated with your weight and the number of drinks that would have been drunk during a certain time period. One drink equals 12 ounces of beer, or 5 ounces of wine, or 1½ ounces of 80–100 proof whiskey.

4. Write down the blood alcohol level from

5. Write down the total number of minutes that would have elapsed between starting to drink and leaving the party, e.g., two hours or 120 minutes.

6. The liver is continuously metabolizing alcohol so we have to make a subtraction from the blood alcohol level from the chart depending upon how long we have been drinking. The correction factor is calculated by first dividing the total number of drinking minutes into 40 minute segments and then multiplying that answer by .01%. This is the correction factor for the alcohol that is metabolized by the liver.

7. Subtract the correction figure from the blood alcohol level that we obtained from the chart in step three. This is the approximate

blood alcohol level after a certain number of drinks in a certain time period.

8. Refer to the chart to see what the effects of this blood alcohol level might be.

The following example illustrates the steps.

A 180-pound person consumes 4 drinks in two hours.

Steps 3 & 4: .083 blood alcohol level from the chart.

Step 5: 2 hours = 120 minutes.

Step 6: (a) $\dfrac{\text{total \# of drinking minutes}}{40 \text{ minutes}} = a$

$a = \dfrac{120 \text{ minutes}}{40} = 3$

(b) a × .01% = correction figure for liver metabolism of alcohol
3 × .01% = .03%

Step 7:　.083　blood alcohol level from the chart
− .030　correction for liver metabolism for alcohol
_____
.053　estimated blood alcohol level for 180-pound person drinking 4 drinks in 2 hours.

Step 8: The chart indicates that at .05 driving becomes increasingly dangerous.

This activity has been used in the classroom and was also set up as a booth for a campus-wide alcohol awareness day. The students found this a meaningful way to estimate how many drinks they could have and the relationship this would have to their blood alcohol level.

Blood alcohol levels (percentage)

Body Weights	1	2	3	4	5	6	7	8	9	10	11	12
100 lbs.	.038	.075	.113	.150	.188	.225	.263	.300	.338	.375	.413	.450
120 lbs.	.031	.063	.094	.125	.156	.188	.219	.250	.281	.313	.344	.375
140 lbs.	.027	.054	.080	.107	.134	.161	.188	.214	.241	.268	.295	.321
160 lbs.	.023	.047	.070	.094	.117	.141	.164	.188	.211	.234	.258	.281
180 lbs.	.021	.042	.063	.083	.104	.125	.146	.167	.188	.208	.229	.250
200 lbs.	.019	.038	.056	.075	.094	.113	.131	.150	.169	.188	.206	.225
220 lbs.	.017	.034	.051	.068	.085	.102	.119	.136	.153	.170	.188	.205
240 lbs.	.016	.031	.047	.063	.078	.094	.109	.125	.141	.156	.172	.188

Drinks[a]

Under .05	.05 to 0.10	.10 to .15	Over .15
Driving is not seriously impaired (although some research indicates fine motor skills may be impaired at .02 or .03 level)	Driving becomes increasingly dangerous .08 is legally drunk in Utah	Driving is dangerous Legally drunk in most states	Driving is very dangerous Legally drunk in any state

[a]One drink equals 1 ounce of 80–100 proof liquor or 12 ounces of beer or 5 ounces of wine.
Reference: New Jersey Department of Law and Public Safety, Division of Motor Vehicles, Trenton, New Jersey.

Senator Hogwash

MICHAEL YOUNG is at Auburn University, Auburn, Alabama 36830.

With a little imagination educational games and activities can be used to promote learning that does get students involved. The objective of one activity may be to introduce factual information while another may promote discussion or enhance decision-making skills. Whatever the overall objective, educational games and learning activities can provide ways to make learning fun. A simulation game designed especially for smoking education is "Senator Hogwash and his tobacco advisory committee."

Simulation games can be used to help clarify values or to introduce factual information along with examining attitudes and/or behaviors about a certain issue. "Senator Hogwash" can bring out not only the health hazards of smoking but can also show that there are many economic, social, and political forces that make quick elimination of cigarette smoking unlikely.

Game Overview

Senator Hogwash is head of the Senate Committee on the Future of Tobacco. To obtain citizen input, and make points with the folks back home, he has appointed a citizen's advisory committee to make recommendations to the Senate Committee. The committee members discuss the issues from the perspective of their assigned roles and prepare a verbal report.

Committee Members

Senator I. M. Hogwash—From Horse Kiss, Kentucky, the Senator serves as an "advisor" to the advisory committee. He has heard ugly rumors of the health hazards of tobacco. He knows that tobacco means money to Kentucky and other tobacco states. He wants to do what is best for all the people he represents but is unclear as to what his position should be.

Medical Doctor—The good doctor once smoked two packs a day but quit smoking about a year ago. He has kicked the habit for good, he hopes. He hates to see anyone smoke because of the craving for a cigarette he still gets whenever he sees someone light up.

Tobacco Company Executive—As vice president of Brown and Jones tobacco company this committee member believes the claims of health hazards due to smoking are unproven. He is not really concerned with health anyway, but with promoting tobacco sales. He believes that government interference in this area would be a blow to the entire free enterprise system of our nation.

Satisfied Smoker—This smoker enjoys his cigarettes and has no desire to quit. He proclaims that smoking is a fundamental right guaranteed by the Constitution and wishes that folks would just let him smoke in peace. He feels that smoking is probably not bad for his health, but even if it is harmful, everyone has to die from something.

Tobacco Farmer—Since tobacco provides this farmer with a major part of his income he is vitally concerned with government plans in this area. He would like to see price supports and other government programs increased. He would hate to see anti-tobacco legislation passed. If that is what the future holds, however, he hopes marijuana will be legalized so he will have another cash crop to take tobacco's place.

Nonsmoker's Rights Advocate—A nonsmoker whose father recently died of lung cancer, this man has led the fight for nonsmoker's rights. He is completely against all forms of smoking and feels some type of government intervention is necessary.

Public Health Educator—This health educator, a specialist in smoking and health, knows the hazards of smoking and is making every effort to turn us into a nation of nonsmokers. He is for higher taxes on cigarettes and feels the funds raised should be earmarked for smoking education and research.

How to Play

The instructor assigns students to play the roles of various committee members. Senator Hogwash, played by the instructor or a student, introduces committee members to each other (players may want to wear name tags) and outlines the committee's task. The committee members discuss the various aspects of the tobacco issue (health hazards, smokers and nonsmokers' rights, economic impact of a possible tobacco prohibition, government's role in tobacco research and promotion, etc.) from the perspective of their assigned roles. Committee members may

compromise when necessary but they try to push through their own ideals whenever possible in order to develop recommendations for the future of tobacco in the United States.

Options

Students not assigned a committee role may be members of the interested public attending the committee meeting. They may wish to ask questions of the Senator and members of the advisory committee. The instructor may wish to appoint more than one advisory committee. These groups could present their recommendations, which may be quite different from group to group. Students who are not members of an advisory committee may be designated Senators and appointed to the Senate Committee on the Future of Tobacco. Advisory committees could present their recommendations to the Senate Committee. Senators could then discuss which recommendations they would like to see incorporated into future legislation.

Students should be introduced to the health aspects of smoking and other issues through lecture material and/or reading assignments. They should not be expected to begin play "cold." Following play, which could run from 30 minutes to one hour or more depending upon the teacher and student interest, a teacher directed discussion period can be of value in providing comments on game play and in restating major issues.

Addictive Behaviors

Student-to-Student Teaching About Tobacco Smoking

Lorraine J. Henke is a health educator at the Eugene Burroughs Junior High School, Accokeek, Maryland.

For the past three years, the decision to smoke or not to smoke has been the subject of formal discussions between eighth grade health education students from Eugene Burroughs Junior High School and elementary students in the fifth and sixth grades in various schools of Prince George's County, Maryland. The project was designed to explore the impact of presenting the smoking aspect of health education between students of close age groups. The assumption was that the fifth and sixth grade students would enthusiastically accept and comprehend the presentation and interchange of health education information with their junior high school student contemporaries. This assumption was proven to be valid.

A typical student-to-student teaching experience consists of a group of seven or eight junior high school health education students visiting a fifth or sixth grade class (frequently a science class). The eighth grade students first present the facts of smoking as a panel, then each of them leads a small group of elementary students in a discussion about the decision to smoke or not to smoke.

During the panel presentation, the junior high school students discuss the effects of tobacco smoking on the body utilizing a machine (constructed by the students) which simulates the effects on the human respiratory system. A filter tip and nonfilter tip cigarette are both "smoked" by the machine. The tar from each of the cigarettes is passed through hollow glass rods representing a person's mouth and throat. The tar that did not adhere to the glass rods then travels to glass test tubes constructed to represent a person's lungs. The presence of tar is always clearly visible, enabling succinct comparisons of tar content to be made between the cigarettes, along with analyses of tar content regardless of the type

of cigarette. Safety precautions to prevent tobacco smoking related fires, why people smoke, and how to quit smoking are presented. The audience is encouraged to join in the discussion and to ask questions of the panel members.

Following the panel presentation, the elementary students are divided into groups and each eighth grader leads a group in discussing the advantages and disadvantages of tobacco smoking. During these discussions, the eighth graders encourage the elementary students to ask questions, to voice honest opinions, and to continue to keep up-to-date regarding the facts about tobacco smoking.

At the conclusion of each instruction program, the visiting junior high school students distribute leaflets stating the facts about tobacco smoking. These leaflets are contributed by the American Cancer Society, the Tuberculosis and Respiratory Disease Association, and the U.S. Department of Health, Education, and Welfare. Also contributed by these organizations for use in the presentations are posters, research data, and other printed materials on tobacco smoking, including the booklet from HEW explaining how to construct the machine which the students used in their presentation.

Several points of interest, noted over the few years of being involved with the student-to-student teaching program, are as follows:

1. Elementary students who plan to attend the junior high school represented by the panel group respond more enthusiastically than do those who are not going to attend that school. Following this revelation, we have encouraged elementary schools to seek the services of the junior high school their students expect to attend.

2. Presentations made to large groups (over 50) of elementary students are not as successful as those given to smaller groups. There appears to be less satisfaction for both

Eighth graders make effective teachers for sixth graders—and especially when they come from the junior high school their audience will attend, when there is a good mix of race, sex, and personality.

the junior high school student teachers and the elementary school students.

3. When the make-up of the panel of junior high students includes a variety of students (in regard to sex, race, personality, and academic achievements), there appears to be a higher audience response (a very good rapport) than if these characteristics were not represented by the junior high school student teachers.

4. Parents of both the elementary and junior high school students involved in the student-to-student teaching program have responded to this form of health education in a very favorable manner.

5. Junior high school students involved in the program have repeatedly stated that their experience in teaching the facts about tobacco smoking has reinforced their decision not to smoke.

6. Repeated requests from the elementary schools have been made to initiate a similar program for other aspects of health education, especially drug education.

Where do we go from here? We are constantly seeking other effective teaching aids like the smoking machine in an attempt to improve our presentations. We are investigating the student-to-student teaching of other aspects of health education. The eighth grade student teachers are invited back each year to relate their experiences regarding tobacco smoking as they progress into the higher school grades. We seek and evaluate the suggestions of the elementary students and their junior high school student teachers. Most important, since the program has been going on for the past few years, we have been able to ask the eighth grade health students (who a few years ago were elementary students attending our student-to-student discussions) what effect the discussions had on their health attitudes and behavior. At this point sufficient data to make a conclusion have not been collected and analyzed. The favorable responses received from those students who had attended the student-to-student discussions, however, please us and spur us on to continue and improve.

The Smoking Game

Ian Newman is associate professor and chairman, Division of Community Health Education, at the University of Nebraska, Lincoln.

In 1964 a new rationale was published to justify an old ethic. The surgeon general's report on smoking and health reinforced the school's position that it should not allow youngsters to smoke in the school building or on the school grounds. Schools had traditionally forbidden smoking, but now they had new medical evidence to support their nonsmoking stand. Needless to say, smoking did not disappear from the high school, junior high school, or even the elementary school. In an attempt to examine the school's traditional stand on cigarette smoking by its students, a long-term examination was made to document the actual smoking behavior conducted within the school. This paper describes something of the behavior of the young people who smoked in the school and the teachers who attempted to prevent their smoking. Information presented here is based on data gathered over a nine-month period of intensive participant observation.

The General Setting of the Game

The events described in this paper took place in a Midwestern junior high school with 1,800 students. It was assumed that while this school was unique, it did have many aspects in common with other schools across the country and the students were, in fact, typical. The school in question was traditional and authoritarian. Discipline was seen as a necessary requirement of efficient administration.

At the time of the study on which this report is based, an important characteristic that distinguished the act of smoking among junior high

* This material was originally presented to the workshop on educational programs influencing youth at the National Conference on Smoking and Health, September 9, 1970, San Diego, California. The work on which this paper is based was performed pursuant to Contract number PH 108-66-192 of the United States Public Health Service, Department of Health, Education, and Welfare; William H. Creswell, Jr., principal investigator; Warren J. Huffman and Donald B. Stone, research associates.

school pupils from smoking among the adult population was its illegality. As one student put it, "When the teachers can't see the kids, the kids smoke and when the kids can't see the teachers, the teachers smoke." This situation was further complicated by the fact that machines dispensed cigarettes to any consumer, regardless of age. Advertising enhanced the pleasures of smoking through subtle inferences. Adults openly violated No Smoking signs and ordinances. Even members of the Board of Education disregarded the many No Smoking signs posted on the walls of their conference room.

At school the rules against smoking applied only to the students. Faculty members smoked in staff rooms and in the locker room office. The school appeared to be the only place where smoking was prohibited only for minors. Students saw this as a clear contradiction of principle. They pointed out, however, that smoking was not the only item of inconsistence. School regulation applying to the length of hair, the color of girls hair, the length of skirts, and the behavior of athletes all represented inconsistencies of various types clearly noted and described by many of the students. With these conditions existing, any action on the part of the students appeared to them to be justified, and activities related to cigarette smoking took on all the dimensions of a game. Smokers played the game of attempting to outsmart the teachers, who for their part attempted to enforce the school's rules and apprehend the smoking students. Achievement in either role was interpreted as winning.

The Contestants—Students

While smoking patterns differed with each subject, there appeared to be a general configuration which characterized the regular ninth-grade smoker. This is illustrated by the following statement recorded during the course of the study.

> After my dad goes to work I usually have one cigarette, then another one on the way to school. You can usually get one more outside the building before you come in and then after second hour you can get at least half a one if you hurry in the washroom upstairs. At lunch time I usually have one outside and then after fifth hour I have

another one. There's usually a bunch of us who go to the washrooms and there's always someone who's willing to stand watch for the teachers.

The Contestants—Teachers

Smoking was illegal for students. Students were encouraged to be like adults. However, when youngsters smoked—like adults—the heavy hand of the school authority descended on them. It was difficult for students to see why 40% of their adult faculty could smoke and they could not. Teachers, both smokers and nonsmokers, thought it their duty to apprehend students who smoked. Students were better at avoiding the teachers than the teachers were at catching the students. The harder the school authorities tried to catch the smokers, the more fun it was for the smokers, and the higher the status one achieved by foiling the authorities' attempt to apprehend.

This set the ground rules for the game. The risks were challenging. The payoff increased with the teachers' increased efforts to catch the cigarette smokers. The teachers felt great frustration. "If only we could cut down a few trees, they'd have no place to hide and we could catch them," lamented one counselor.

The reward to the students was expressed by one nonsmoker, who said:

> You know, I get a kick out of it every time I see a kid smoke and get away with it. It seems there are still a few things around here that you can do and get away with. It's good to know we can still beat the teachers.

Strategies of the Game

Subjects and other informants reported that smoking occasionally took place in the locker rooms, shower rooms, industrial arts shops, photographic dark room, and even in the classrooms. However, the majority of smoking in this particular school was limited to the washrooms and to a specific location adjacent to the school entrance but hidden from view by four small trees. Because both of these locations were essentially within range of easy scrutiny by the faculty, numerous techniques were utilized to foil detection. Description of one of these will serve to illustrate the process of the game.

The majority of the smoking in the school building was done during the lunch hour and between class periods. At lunch time students went to the cafeteria in three shifts. During lunch they were restricted to an area including the cafeteria and the hallways immediately adjacent to it. This area included boys and girls washrooms, which became the centers for smoking activity. Because this location was heavily traveled by faculty going

to and from lunch, smoking required a well-coordinated team effort. To further complicate the matter for the smokers, two counselors were assigned to patrol this general area.

Those concerned about being caught posted "guards" outside the washroom to warn of approaching faculty members. Methods utilized by the guards to convey their warnings varied with the urgency of the situation. The simplest method was for the guard to go inside and tell the smokers that someone was approaching. However, this endangered the guard as he then ran the risk of being caught in the smoking setting. Another procedure employed by the guard was simply to kick the door with his heel to warn of the approaching faculty member. Still another variation of this procedure was to kick the radiator pipe which passed through the wall. On occasions when a teacher approached too rapidly, or was unnoticed until the last moment, the student on guard would open the door for the teacher and greet him by name in a loud voice so that those inside would get the warning. Nonsmokers often acted as guards, and it was reported that it was safer to have a nonsmoker stand watch. They were less likely to leave their posts for a few puffs with the rest of the group.

Inside the washroom the smokers took additional precautions to avoid being caught. It was a common practice for them to stand close to urinals, sinks, or toilet stools while smoking so that it was an easy matter to get rid of the cigarettes. A wet paper towel was often kept ready to snuff out the cigarette as a last resort to avoid being caught if a teacher entered. Smokers would often stand on the toilet stools which enabled them to exhale smoke close to the air exhaust ducts on the wall. This cleared the smoke from the room. This also provided for easy disposal of cigarette butts by flushing them down the toilet.

While it was not possible to observe the smoking behavior of the girls as closely, informants reported similar practices in their washrooms; however, fewer girls smoked and the necessity for an elaborate warning system was less important. While as many as fifteen boys might congregate to smoke cigarettes at any one time, it was unusual for more than five girls to be present in a smoking situation. Girls were more likely to smoke alone or with one or two classmates. They were more apt to smoke when the washroom was empty or they avoided smoking in school altogether.

Smoking outside the school building, but on the school grounds, was less hazardous. But again students developed sophisticated systems to avoid detection. The most popular location, adjacent to the front entrance of the school and behind a group of small trees, often produced a two-step communication system to foil teachers' attempts to apprehend smokers in the act.

Students found numerous ways to test their skills of concealment against the teachers' skills of detection. Students would smoke in the front rows of the school movie theater on recreation nights. They smoked in the industrial arts shops where numerous odors aided in concealment and in shower and locker rooms which were usually unsupervised. On occasion, when faculty members supervised the loading of school buses, smokers would approach the supervising teacher to see how close they could get without being caught. Smokers and their friends appeared to enjoy the success of such endeavors.

Chances of Changing the Game Plan

Throughout the year the game varied in intensity. At times the faculty would win out, several smokers would be caught and suspended, and smoking would appear to subside. This reinforced the faculty's feeling that discipline did solve the problem. In reality, the smokers had been forced to regroup and utilize their most successful strategies. For awhile they were more careful and worked harder in maintaining the covert nature of their smoking behavior.

As in any game, learning took place. Students decided on new ploys to outsmart teachers and at times they even chose to quit the game completely; they became nonsmokers. However, to change roles and become a nonsmoker was difficult.

Teachers seemed to react to smokers the same way they reacted to students who were failing academically, probably because they had observed that smoking and failing were often associated. Students who were grouped into either of these two categories tended to be treated differently by most teachers. On teachers' evaluations, for example, smokers were rated lower than their nonsmoking colleagues. Teachers expected less of these students and tended to be suspicious of them. As a result, students who were smokers tended to be offered little latitude within the school. By comparison, nonsmokers who functioned successfully within the school were given considerable freedom, which they often abused.

As one individual, a class monitor and football team member, stated:

I know,. I can do just about anything I please around here. I get on real good with the teachers. I can walk the halls whenever I want. Teachers let me out of class, monitors never ask me for my pass; if they do, I just tell them so-and-so sent me on an errand and they never report me for not having a pass—it's rather bad actually.

By contrast, a student who was both a smoker and a poor student related the following incident. He had been given a signed hall pass to visit the office. However, he was apprehended on his way and finally escorted to his office by an assistant principal and a teacher, both of whom questioned the authenticity of his pass. The student's explanation was as follows:

I gave my pass to the teacher and he made some crack about getting out of his class—he's a good guy, however, you know. Then, as I was walking down the hall (this teacher) comes out of his classroom and asks me for my pass. I shows it to him and he makes some wise crack about forging it. He's always sticking his nose where it's not wanted. Then, I goes to the washroom and I came out and (another teacher) asks for my pass. He says the pass was not for the toilet and that I shouldn't waste time. Just as I came in the door, I stopped for a drink of water and she takes my pass and says it don't look like your writing. I gave her a bit of lip and whamo, the assistant principal appears.

These incidents and others suggest that teachers' attitudes toward certain students became inflexible. Consequently, any attempt by these students to modify their own behavioral game plan was met with little recognition and considerable resistance. As one male smoker said:

I decided I was going to go good this year. I even quit smoking. I tried real hard, but they (the teachers) just wouldn't give me a chance. I gave up in the end . . . it seemed that whenever there was trouble they thought I was involved and even when I wasn't they just wouldn't let me be good.

The Observer's Perspective

Having watched the game from the vantage point of a participant observer, trusted by the students and the teachers and not required to take sides in the contest, I noted several points over the duration of the year.

1. Cigarette smoking was not an end in itself. At this age, it wasn't the taste or the association with coffee that encouraged the students to smoke. Smoking was, in fact, just a symptom of the larger problem. The majority of nonsmoking kids thought their friends smoked to "be big" or to achieve status. Smokers didn't admit to this, although their actions tended to confirm the motivating forces of status, or at least compensatory behavior.

2. Records showed that young people who smoked at this early age were similar in IQ to

their nonsmoking contemporaries. While the smokers knew what was expected of them, they also knew that they were often not meeting these expectations. School records showed that they were correct in their recognition of low achievement. They were more likely to be failing courses, truant, tardy, and suspended from school than were their nonsmoking contemporaries. They didn't participate in the extracurricular life of the school and their fellow students tended to see them as low social status individuals. They chose friends who were like themselves for support. In other words, they tended to group together as a team—the peer group team.

3. Teachers tended to type individuals who smoked and held lower expectations for them. As a result, teachers tended to resist changes in behavior on the part of the smoker. Smokers had great difficulty in casting off the smoking image of low achievement and poor behavior if they chose to quit smoking.

4. As with all games, one left the scene of contest wondering what would happen if other strategies had been employed by the contestants. It appeared that the smokers had read the wrong signals. While they still attended school, they had already dropped out. The school had provided them with few rewards and they looked other places, in other contests, for more meaningful rewards.

What would have happened if the school had stopped harassing the smokers and admitted to its own hypocrisy, thereby removing the payoff from the game? If at the same time there had been alternative and meaningful activities available to the smokers would they have found less encouragement to smoke?

Would new courses, interesting courses that appealed to these early dropouts, have recaptured their restless spirits to a point where they would have at least become a part of the educational process?

What new methods could be used and what new ways could be made available to these young smokers to find status within the system rather than being forced to compete for status in the smoking game?

How many poorly planned anti-smoking education campaigns actually enhance the status of the smoker by putting him in a position of brave risk taker—willing to stand fast against the statistics, the true games player—willing to gamble against odds and possibly win?

Smoking has to be recognized as something more than a dirty habit. It was a practice, complex and multidimensional in nature, even for the junior high school student. Unfortunately, however, it appeared that the teachers had overlooked this fact and thought they could win out with a single strategy of firm discipline. It was apparent that this single strategy game plan was not successful.

Addictive Behaviors

Making Tobacco Education Relevant

To the School-Age Child

John R. Seffrin, is professor and chairman of Health and Safety Education and director of Operation SmART at Indiana University, Bloomington, IN 47405.

School health education is faced today with a number of challenging opportunities to improve the quality of life through effective instructional programs. Whether it's sexually transmitted diseases, suicide, teenage drinking, illegitimacy or accidental deaths, most health educators feel that our discipline can and should help ameliorate these health problems through sound school health education programs.

Probably no greater challenge exists for school health education today than that of cigarette smoking among youth. Although the per capita consumption of cigarettes has dropped during the last three years, the estimated health-care cost to society because of cigarette-induced illness is fifteen billion dollars annually.[1] What is more important is that at least 340,000 Americans die each year prematurely because they smoke cigarettes.[2] In the words of Joseph A. Califano, former Secretary of Health, Education and Welfare, the unadorned facts clearly show that cigarette smoking is "public health enemy number one."

The cigarette smoking dilemma is a complex cultural problem with many interacting personal and social forces. However, the gross figures suggest strongly that the school curriculum has failed to prevent children and teenagers from beginning to smoke. For example, although the percentage of adults who smoke has gradually declined since 1964, the percentage of children and teenagers who smoke has increased. The rate of increase among teenage girls is particularly alarming.[3] All told, today six million children and teenagers smoke.[4] Past research and experience clearly show that 1) the majority of these youngsters will continue to smoke regularly for life; and, 2) they will be less well and their lives shorter because of their smoking habit.[5,6]

Finally, since the decision to smoke or not to smoke is made very early in life (almost always before age twenty and often by junior high school), the role of school health education, particularly during the primary and middle school years, is of critical importance if health educators are to reach students before they start smoking.[7,8] Until and unless comprehensive efforts are made to provide each school child with meaningful health instruction regarding cigarettes, the carnage in human health and life is likely to continue.

Personal Choice and Responsibility

Effectiveness of instruction is more related to how we teach than to what we teach. In the area of personal lifestyle it is important for the health educator to recognize the pluralism in our society. With the contemporary emphasis placed on personal rights and values, instructional strategies should be tailored accordingly. Therefore, careful planning by the teacher is necessary to provide a balanced as well as scientifically accurate instructional program. For example, in addition to teaching about the health consequences of smoking, instructional time should be used to explore the reasons why some people choose to smoke. In short, the teacher should develop an objective atmosphere in which the pros and cons of smoking can be fully explored.

The theme should be: the student has the ultimate responsibility to decide whether or not to smoke; therefore, the student must be given the pertinent facts in an objective setting. The goal is to provide the student with an opportunity to make a decision based on facts and personal values. Attendant to this approach is the accompanying need for the student to accept responsibility for his or her decision. In an effort to develop an awareness of the full responsibility involved in such a decision, instructional time should be given to explore a number of social issues such as accuracy in advertising, special insurance rates for smokers, and non-smokers' rights.

In the past many working education efforts have been restricted to a narrow, one-sided, health-facts unit which could be accurately described as a "thou shalt not" approach. Besides being a "turn-off" for many students, its greatest weakness was that, in omitting substantive socio-political issues, some of the strong persuasions against taking up smoking were never developed. Thus, millions of children and teenagers have decided to smoke, at least in part, because the only disincentive was an obscure threat to their health decades in the future. To be truly responsive to student needs and to maximize the relevancy and potential impact of our teaching, we must go beyond the statistical correlations associating smoking with age-onset diseases. Morbidity and mortality figures and facts are not enough.

Suggested Facts and Concepts

With the knowledge explosion it is impossible to teach all the facts in any area; thus the professional responsibility of the teacher to select appropriate information to develop valid concepts is critical. Following are selected examples of content and concepts which can be made relevant to students.

Cigarette smoking is our nation's leading preventable health problem. Consensus exists among medical scientists that cigarette smoking is the greatest cause of preventable illness and premature death in the United States.[9,10] This year, for example, over 122,000 people will develop lung cancer in the United States; at least 80% of these cases are due to cigarette smoking.[11] Additionally, thousands more will develop cancers of the throat, oral cavity, pancreas, esophagus and urinary bladder because they smoke.[12,13] Heart diseases, our nation's leading cause of death, will take the lives of smokers at least twice as frequently as non-smokers.[14] Chronic obstructive lung disease, one of our nation's fastest-growing chronic diseases, is largely caused by cigarette smoking.[15] In short, after 30,000 scientific studies over three decades it is apparent that not one measure in preventive medicine could

Photo: National Cancer Institute, *Smoking Programs for Youth*

do more to improve health and to prevent premature death than the control of cigarette smoking.[16]

Cigarette smoking is deleterious to your health now. The association of cigarette smoking to the aforementioned diseases is well established and widely recognized. However, less well known is that cigarette smoking is harmful to the smoker's health immediately. The adverse effects of smoking begin with the first cigarette and get progressively worse as smoking continues.[17] Immediate negative physiological responses to the smoker include increased heart rate, elevated blood pressure, constriction of blood vessels and trachial irritation.[18,19] While permanent, irreversible damage to the lungs does not occur immediately, hyperplasia (overgrowth of cells and overproduction of mucous) begins within weeks of regular cigarette smoking.[20,21] Ciliary action is damaged and trachial-mucosal velocity (TMV) is reduced while one smokes.[22,23] This, in part, explains why smokers are more prone to infectious diseases of the respiratory tract.[24]

In recent years, studies have shown basic pulmonary dysfunction in teenagers who have smoked for only a few years.[25] Although some of the harmful effects of smoking are reversible if a person quits in time (e.g. smokers' lung cancer mortality rates return to non-smoker rates 10 to 15 years after smoking ceases),[26] lung and respiratory tract tissue damage begins with the onset of smoking and becomes worse the longer one smokes.[27] Some scar tissue will re-

sult after only a few months of regular smoking.[28]

There is no such thing as safe smoking. Occasionally reports on smoking suggest that "moderate" or "light" smoking of low tar and nicotine cigarettes may be safe. This implication arises from the well-established fact that smoking's impact on health is a dose/response phenomenon.[29] The number of cigarettes smoked, the frequency of puffing, and the depth of the inhale all relate to increased risks.[30]

The inference, however, that there may be a safe or threshold level below which no harm occurs is unsubstantiated and invalid.[31,32] As already pointed out, adverse effects begin early and grow progressively worse over time.[33] Further, although low tar and nicotine cigarettes are assumed to be less hazardous, no evidence exists which would indicate that they are safe. On the contrary, certain harmful substances, such as carbon monoxide, are in greater concentration in the low tar and low nicotine brands.[34] Scientifically, it is very difficult to make blanket statements about the relative risks of different brands because of individual differences in smoking technique. For example, some smokers who switch to a low tar and nicotine brand may draw harder or inhale deeper and smoke more cigarettes; thus, the relative dosage of nicotine and other substances may be about the same as before.

In conclusion, if a person must smoke, a low tar and nicotine cigarette

may be the least harmful; however, from a health vantage point, any smoking is hazardous to one's health.

Cigarette smoking can be harmful to others, and especially to fetuses. In addition to the well-known irritation factor, which at least 60% of all people experience, there are real health threats from exposure to second-hand smoke.[35,36] The most alarming threat is to persons who are already chronically ill with diseases like coronary artery disease, bronchitis, and chronic obstructive pulmonary disease.[37] For example, people with existing heart disease will develop angina pectoris (chest pain) upon exertion sooner when breathing air polluted with tobacco smoke.[38] Further, animal studies have shown significantly more malignant tumors among those animals breathing second-hand smoke on a daily basis.[39] Finally, children exposed regularly to cigarette smoke have twice the respiratory disease rate of other children.[40] Although the smoker is affected most by smoking, the non-smoker who breathes air polluted with cigarette smoke does experience untoward physiological effects.[41] These unhealthy and immediate effects include elevated blood pressure, increased heart rate, and abnormal carboxyhemaglobin levels (carbon monoxide in the blood).[42] Recent studies confirm that even healthy adults develop marked small-airways dysfunction from breathing secondhand smoke.[43]

The most fearsome impact of second-hand smoke may be on the fetus of the pregnant smoker. Unless the mother stops smoking before the fourth month of pregnancy, some untoward effect can be expected in the baby.[44] Since carbon monoxide crosses the placental bearier, the unborn fetus can be expected to develop carboxyhemoglobin levels comparable to the mother's.[45,46] Since it is known that carbon monoxide displaces oxygen in the blood, it is obvious that the fetus is put at a distinct disadvantage during the most important period of its growth and development. For example, the human fetus' brain is growing at the rate of one to two milligrams per minute at the time of delivery.[47] Thus, any oxygen deprivation is most critical. In addition to having more miscarriages and stillbirths, smoking mothers have babies who weigh less at birth; also their babies are more apt to die during the first year after birth; and, their babies have more respiratory disease during childhood and adolescence.[48,49] One of the most discouraging findings educationally has been the discovery that children whose mothers smoked during pregnancy do poorer on achievement tests in math and reading at ages 7 and 11.[50]

Regular cigarette smoking usually results in a serious dependency problem. Like any drug of abuse, tobacco has the potential of causing serious dependency. Unlike users of other drugs of abuse, however, research indicates that tobacco users will usually become dependent for life—they will be less well and their lives shorter because of their smoking.[51] For example, it is estimated that about 10-15% of the people alive today who ever used heroin are still dependent on it. However, 66% of those still alive who ever smoked cigarettes are currently still dependent on cigarettes and smoke them daily.[52]

While research to elucidate the mechanisms of dependency continues, it is safe to say that cigarette smoking can and usually does result in strong dependency. The psychological factors associated with habit formation and desire to smoke seem to be paramount; but, at least for some smokers, the development of a physical dependence to nicotine may also occur.[53] These stark facts should be included in educational units so that those deciding to smoke are aware, in advance, of the likelihood of future dependency. It is known from national polls that at least 8 in 10 smokers would like to quit if there were an easy way. Such information is particularly critical in view of the recent trend in children experimenting with tobacco at earlier ages. A 1967 British survey of teenagers indicated that among those who smoked more than one cigarette, 80% ultimately became regular smokers.[55]

The advantages of not smoking far outweigh the advantages of smoking. Children and teenagers who choose to smoke do so for certain reasons. Although these reasons may not be clearly elucidated and evaluated, and just as importantly, they may not be understood by the smoker, we must acknowledge that all behavior, healthy as well as unhealthy, is caused. It is a logical assumption that many smokers find their habit enjoyable and somehow, reinforcing. For some youngsters, smoking may provide a way of emulating adults; for others a way of rebelling; and for still others, simply a satisfaction of curiosity.[56,57] Educators should explore with their students these and other possible reasons for smoking. In so doing, educators should avoid a condescending attitude toward reasons advanced in favor of smoking. Since one's values relate intimately to one's rationale for behavior, it is inappropriate to label reasons as right or wrong. The merits and demerits of various reasons should be explored in an atmosphere of respect with an emphasis on value clarification.

However, any comprehensive analysis of the pros and cons associated with smoking leads to one very critical conclusion; that is, the advantages of not smoking far outweigh the advantages of smoking.

Issues for Class Discussion

Since the decision to smoke or not to smoke is an individual one, much of the educational strategy should focus on personalizing lessons. As stated, there should be adequate coverage of the various values and motivations involved in choosing a course of action.

However, to stop at the personal level would be remiss in light of the health care dilemma facing society today. In an effort to explore the responsibility of the individual in society, a careful examination of social policies regarding cigarette smoking is important and relevant. Three examples follow of critical socio-political issues which should be dealt with in the secondary curriculum.

What should be our federal policy toward tobacco? Currently the federal government is inconsistent and contradictory in its policy toward tobacco. Simultaneously, two cabinet-level departments pursue policies which have antithetical objectives. The Department of Agriculture (USDA) continues to support and promote tobacco production. In 1977, for example, the U.S. Department of Agriculture spent approximately 65 million dollars on the various aspects of administering the price-support program for tobacco.[58] Further, the nation's lawmakers included tobacco in Public Law 480, the "Food for Peace" program.[59] Under this program millions of dollars in tobacco have been sent to developing countries around the world.

On the other hand, the U.S. Department of Health and Human Services (DHHS) continues to battle cigarette smoking in many ways. In 1964 the first and landmark *Surgeon General's Report on Smoking* was published. Since then a number of efforts have been instituted at the national level to combat smoking through school and public health education. In 1978, DHEW Secretary Califano established the Office on

Photo: National Cancer Institute, *Smoking Programs for Youth*

Smoking and Health, and money continues to be spent on anti-smoking programs.[60]

Who should pay the smoker's health care bill? The cost of medical care in America continues to rise even faster than the inflation rate. This year, Americans will spend over 245 billion dollars on personal health services, more than any other nation in the

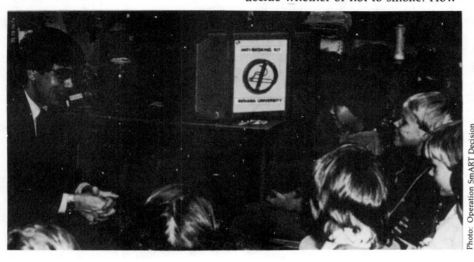

Photo: Operation SmART Decision

world.[61] With the trend toward some form of prepaid, social-health insurance plan for all, greater emphasis needs to be placed on the prevention of disease. For example, it is estimated that 350,000 people will die this year from diseases caused by cigarette smoking.[62] Prior to their death many incurred large medical bills resulting from expensive treatment and lengthy stays in hospitals. Current estimates are that each year at least seven billion dollars are spent on the direct medical costs of treating diseases caused by cigarette smoking. If one adds the lost productivity, the total cost jumps to a staggering 20 billion dollars annually.[63] Presently, the direct health costs are borne primarily by private insurance companies. Eventually, they may all be paid through national health insurance. Regardless of the system, private or governmental, the consumer pays—all the consumers. Should nonsmokers pay as much in premiums or taxes as the smoker?

What are the rights of smokers and non-smokers? The spirit of this age is *rights:* rights for the handicapped, rights for Blacks, rights for the aged and rights for children. In all of the above examples, one common denominator exists. Each one of the above represents a minority group. In the case of nonsmokers' rights, we are talking about the *majority.* Most children and adults

do not smoke. In spite of this fact, many who are bothered by cigarette smoke feel as though they should not express their discomfort, since it is the smoker's right to smoke.

However, no one is proposing to take away the smoker's right to smoke. On the contrary, all major groups active in the smoking and health controversy maintain that a person has the right to decide whether or not to smoke. However, a distinction needs to be made between a right and a freedom. That is, although one has a right to choose to smoke or not to smoke, one does *not* have the freedom to engage in the practice at will.

Since the beginning of our country, certain limitations have been placed on personal rights. Generally, these limitations are determined by two factors: the health and safety of the public; and the rights that might be abridged by the unrestricted practice of the first right. The adoption of speed limits is an example of protecting public safety. A great jurist once wrote, "My right to swing my fist ends when my fist reaches the end of your nose." Consistent with these principles and precedents, one's right to smoke should not be total and unrestricted. For years, for safety purposes, smoking has been properly disallowed in combustible areas, and, smoking in bed is against the law.

We now know that ambient cigarette smoke can be hazardous to the non-smoker's health, especially to children and persons with chronic illnesses. Since society should promote the public health, a new look at rights for smokers and non-smokers is justified and appropriate.

Summary

Americans consume 615 billion cigarettes annually.[64] Although the per capita consumption for adults has dropped over the past fifteen years, the amount of cigarettes being smoked by children and teenagers has increased. The percent of teenage girls smoking has nearly doubled during the last decade.[65] Because of this trend toward more smoking among the young, and because of smoking's effect on human health and life, educators must redouble their efforts. In spite of the diseases exacted on humans as a result of smoking, cigarette smoking, as such, is not a medical problem; but rather, the real problem lies in educating youngsters prior to the age at which the critical decision to smoke or not to smoke is made.

Through careful planning and professional discretion the school-health team can address this challenge in ways that are meaningful and relevant to students. No longer do we need to threaten the child with dread diseases in the distant future; but rather, instructional strategies can be designed to respect the student's right to choose. However, in choosing, it is imperative that the student grasp the profundity of the decision. Through a comprehensive and balanced instructional effort the student can better understand the personal as well as social ramifications of cigarette smoking. With an emphasis on the role of values and motivations in decision making the student can begin to appreciate the words of Frost:

"Two roads diverged in a wood, and I -
I took the one less traveled by,
And that has made all the difference."[66]

[1]American Cancer Society, Inc. *A national dilemma: cigarette smoking or the health of Americans – report of the National Commission on Smoking and Public Policy to the Board of Directors,* 1978, 4.

[2]U.S. DHEW. Smoking and health, report of the Surgeon General, Washington, DC: USPHS, 1979, ii.

[3]U.S. DHEW. *The smoking digest,* National Cancer Institute, 1977, 13.

[4]Horn, D. How much real progress have we made in the fight against smoking? *Bull Am Lung Assoc,* 1979, 65, 6–9.

[5]Russell, M. A. H. Smoking problems: an overview, in *Research on smoking behavior, National Institute on Drug Abuse Research Monograph 17,* M. E. Jarvik, J. W. Cullen, E. R. Gritz, T. M. Vogt, and L. J. West, (eds.), (U.S. Department of Health, Education and Welfare. Publication No. (ADM) 78-581). Rockville, MD.: National Institute on Drug Abuse, 1977, 13–33.

[6]U.S. DHEW: *The health consequences of smoking, report of the Surgeon General,* Office

on Smoking and Health, 1978.

[7]American School Health Association. *Introducing tobacco education in the elementary school K-4*, Kent, OH: American School Health Association, 1978, 2.

[8]WHO. *Smoking and its effects on health, report of a WHO Expert Committee*, Geneva, Switzerland: World Health Organization, 1975, 29–33.

[9]Fletcher, C. M., & Horn, D. Smoking and health, *WHO Chronicle*, 1970, 24, 345–370.

[10]U.S. DHEW. *The health consequences of smoking*, p. 2.

[11]American Cancer Society, Inc.: *Cancer facts and figures 1981*, New York, NY: American Cancer Society, Inc., 1979, 9, 14.

[12]*Ibid.*, p. 19.

[13]U.S. DHEW: *The health consequences of smoking*, ch. 5.

[14]Steinfeld, J. L. Presentation at Opening Plenary Session of the 3rd World Conference on Smoking and Health, in *Proceedings of the 3rd World Conference on Smoking and Health, II*, J. Steinfeld, W. Griffiths, K. Ball, & R. M. Taylor, (eds.), (U.S. Department of Health, Education and Welfare. Publication No. NIH 77-1414). Washington, D.C.: U.S. Government Printing Office, 1976, 21.

[15]U.S. DHEW. *The health consequences of smoking, 1975*, (Publication No. CDC 76-8704). Washington, D.C.: U.S. Government Printing Office, 1975, 61.

[16]Fletcher, C. M., & Horn, D. Smoking and health.

[17]Worick, W. W., and Schaller, W. E. *Alcohol, tobacco, and drugs*, Englewood Cliffs, NJ: Prentice-Hall, Inc., 1977, 77–109.

[18]*Ibid*

[19]Diehl, H. S. *Tobacco and your health: the smoking controversy*, New York, NY: McGraw-Hill, Inc., 1969, 47–51.

[20]Jay, S. J., Associate Professor of Medicine, Indiana University School of Medicine, Pulmonary Section, interview, February 27, 1979.

[21]*Essentials of life and health*, New York, NY: Random House (CRM Books), 1977, 86–87.

[22]American Lung Association. Chronic smoking lowers rate at which the lungs clear mucus, *Bull Am Lung Assoc.*, July-August, 1977, 15.

[23]Newhouse, M. T. Effect of cigarette smoking on mucociliary clearance, in *Proceedings of the 3rd World Conference on Smoking and Health, II, op. cit.*, pp. 131–137.

[24]Diehl, Tobacco and your health, 87–95.

[25]U.S. DHEW, *The health consequences of smoking*, 1978, ch. 6.

[26]U.S. DHEW, *The Smoking Digest*, p. 28.

[27]Royal College of Physicians of London: *Smoking or health – the third report from the Royal College of Physicians of London*, Trent, England: Pitman Medical Publishing Co. LTD, 1977, 76–81.

[28]Jay: op. cit.

[29]U.S. DHEW. *Report of the Surgeon General on smoking and health*, 1964 through 1978.

[30]Diehl, Tobacco and your health, p. 202.

[31]*Ibid.*, 201–206.

[32]Royal College of Physicians of London, *Smoking or health*, pp. 121–122.

[33]Worick and Schaller, *Alcohol, tobacco and drugs*.

[34]U.S. DHEW, *The health consequences of smoking*, 1978, ch. 11.

[35]Speer, F. Tobacco and the nonsmoker, *Arch Environ Health*, 1968, 16, 443–446.

[36]Burns, D. M. Consequences of smoking – the involuntary smoker, in *Proceedings of the 3rd World Conference on Smoking and Health, II*, 51–58.

[37]Tate, C. F. The effects of tobacco smoke on the non-smoking cardiopulmonary public, in *Proceedings of the 3rd World Conference on Smoking and Health, II*, 329–335.

[38]Aronow, W. S. Carbon monoxide and cardiovascular disease, in *Proceedings of the 3rd World Conference on Smoking and Health, I*, E. L. Wynder, D. Hoffmann, and G. B. Gori, (eds.). (U.S. Department of Health, Education and Welfare Publication No. NIH 76-1221). Washington, D.C.: U.S. Government Printing Office, 1976, 321–328.

[39]U.S. DHEW: *The health consequences of smoking, a report of the Surgeon General: 1972*, (Publication No. HSM 72-7516). Washington, D.C.: U.S. Government Printing Office, 1972, 121–135.

[40]Colley, J. R. T., et al. Influence of passive smoking and parental phlegm on pneumonia and bronchitis in early childhood, *Lancet*, 1974, II, 1031–1034.

[41]U.S. DHEW: *The health consequences of smoking, 1975*, 87–106.

[42]White, J.R. & Frobe, H.F. Small-airways dysfunction in non-smokers chronically exposed to tobacco smoke. *New England Journal of Medicine*, 1980, 302, 720-723.

[43]Burns, D. M. Consequences of smoking.

[44]Goldstein, H. Smoking in pregnancy: the statistical controversy and its resolution, in *Proceedings of the 3rd World Conference on Smoking and Health, II*, 201–210.

[45]Longo, L. D. The biological effects of carbon monoxide on the pregnant woman, fetus, and newborn infant, *Am J Obstet Gynecol*, 1977, 29, 69–103.

[46]*Ibid*.

[47]Dobbing, J. All flesh is grass, *Kaiser Aluminum News: The World Food Crisis – Man, Mind, Soul*, 1968, 26, p. 13.

[48]Butler, N. R., et al. Cigarette smoking in pregnancy: its influence on birth weight and prenatal mortality, *Br Med J*, 1972, 2, 127–130.

[49]Meyer, M. B., & Tonascia, J. A. Maternal smoking, pregnancy complications and prenatal mortality, *Am J Obstet Gynecol*, 1977, 128, 494–502.

[50]Butler, N. R., & Goldstein, H. Smoking in pregnancy and subsequent child development, *Br Med J*, 1973, 4, 573–575.

[51]U.S. DHEW: *The health consequences of smoking*, 1978, Preface, p. 5, ch. 1, 2, 3, 4, 6.

[52]Blair, G. Why Dick can't stop smoking – the politics behind our national addiction, *Mother Jones*, January 1979, 31–42.

[53]Royal College of Physicians of London; *Smoking or health*, pp. 43–44.

[54]Olshavsky, R. W. *No more butts – a psychologist's approach to quitting cigarettes*, Bloomington, IN.: Indiana University Press, 1977, 3.

[55]Royal College of Physicians of London, *Smoking or health*, p. 89.

[56]U.S. DHEW: *Teenage smoking–national patterns of cigarette smoking, ages 12 through 18, in 1972 and 1974*. (Publication No. NIH 76-931, Public Health Service) 1976.

[57]Seffrin, J. R. Risks, rewards and values, *Health Values*, September/October 1977, 1, 197–199.

[58]Eckholm, Cutting tobacco's toll, p. 19.

[59]*Ibid.*, p. 21.

[60]Califano Jr., J. A. A new commitment to wellness, *Bull Am Lung Assoc.*, November 1978, 64, 5–10.

[61]Health Insurance Institute, *Sourcebook of health insurance data, 1979–1980*, Washington, DC: Health Insurance Institute, 1979, 47.

[62]*Cancer facts and figures, 1981*.

[63]*Ibid.*, p. 2.

[64]*Ibid.*, p. 1.

[65]Hill, H. Situational analysis: women and smoking, in *Proceedings of the 3rd World Conference on Smoking and Health, II*, pp. 291–297.

[66]Frost, R. *Complete poems of Robert Frost*, New York, NY: Holt, Rinehart, and Winston, 1967, 131.

TEACHING IDEAS

Addictive Behaviors

A Humanistic-Individualized Approach to Drug Education

JERRY L. GREENE is an assistant professor and PHILLIP G. HUNTSINGER is an associate professor of health, physical education, and recreation at the University of Kansas, Lawrence, Kansas 66045.

Many teachers individualize instruction to some extent without realizing it by giving special instructions to certain students, by allowing variety in student roles in class, or by allowing work on different skills at different times. This individual attention may be at the expense of the other students because the teacher's plan does not allow for special pacing and involvement. The problem is to create an environment which will let the individual progress through the learning program with a high degree of self-direction and involvement without impeding other students.

The primary objective of the humanistic-individualized approach is to get the students involved in the learning process by doing and thinking with all their capabilities. It is up to the teacher to help students find the most productive way to the student-teacher agreed upon goals. This kind of approach should help students learn the process of self-education in addition to the subject matter.

The following steps should be adhered to for implementing this teaching strategy:

Self-diagnosis: The teacher should develop this part of the instructional unit so that it is conducive to the student's mode of learning. See the diagnosis exercises.

Prescribed activities: The teacher must determine the kind and quantity of input and practice that students must complete before they can meet the desired objectives.

Program of learning experiences: This is the total program of prescribed experiences that the teacher develops for the students. It includes: Input—these experiences allow the students to further develop their competencies in areas shown to be weak by self-diagnosis. Output—these experiences will allow students to demonstrate the skills and knowledge developed in weak areas after strengthening by input experiences.

Evaluation: The students and the teacher can determine if the learning objective has been attained as a result of the input and output experiences by analyzing specific performance objectives developed for the unit.

We used this approach to teach drug education in the sixth grade, but it is easily adaptable to a number of health education topics. In our class of about 30, the children had been exposed to quality health education from grades 1 through 5. The text used throughout the district was the Scott, Foresman series. The four-week unit covered illegal drugs. The legal ones (alcohol, caffeine, nicotine) were studied in other units.

Self-Diagnosis

Directions: Read the questions and mentally answer them. If you believe you know the correct answer put a check in the "yes" column. If you are not sure of the answer or do not know, check the "no" column. If you need to, check the accuracy of your answers by comparing with other students or with the teacher's

notes. If a question was answered incorrectly, change your answer to the appropriate column.

Can you–   YES NO
1. explain what the term "narcotic" means?
2. define the term "hallucinogenic?"
3. explain what the term "depressant" means?
4. identify the meaning associated with a stimulant drug?
4. describe a volatile substance?
6. classify the following drugs: LSD, tranquilizer, heroin, aerosol sprays, "pep pills"?
7. describe how glue sniffing affects the body?
8. describe the difference between the physical effects of stimulants and depressants?
9. explain what effect a narcotic would have on the body?
10. define drug abuse?
11. list ten reasons why people use drugs?
12. identify common household substances that are dangerous to the body?
13. list ten slang terms associated with drugs?

Prescribed Activities

Directions: Determine the number of checks in the "yes" column. Now determine the percentages. To increase your knowledge you may use the suggested program of learning experiences recommended in the Input and Practice columns.

Results	Inputs	Practices
More than 80%	#1, 7, 8	#1, 7
60 to 80%	#1, 3, 7	#1, 5, 6
40 to 60%	#1, 3, 5, 7	#2, 3, 4, 6
Less than 40%	#1, 2, 4, 5, 6, 7	#2, 3, 4, 5, 6

Program of Learning Experiences

Directions: The learner should follow any or all suggestions in this program. All of the experiences are designed to improve ability to motivate students for individualized instruction.

Proposed learning objective: The learner will be able to develop a basic understanding of drugs and drug usage.

Input

1. Read Chapter 6, *Health and Growth: Book 6* (Scott, Foresman series, 1974).
2. Discuss why our culture is called a "pill culture."
3. Read a programmed learning unit on drugs and drug use.
4. Discuss what role age should play in drug use.
5. View the "Inside-Out" film series and discuss.
6. Discuss the scope of the local drug scene.
7. Listen to a speaker from a community organization that specializes in some aspect of drugs.
8. Plan an input of your own.

Practice

1. Write a report on drugs.
2. Collect and post newspaper and magazine stories on drugs.
3. Plan a role playing scene showing how the character Charlie Brown would describe today's drug users.
4. Develop a bulletin board showing dangerous household substances.
5. Make a crossword puzzle using only slang drug terms.
6. Draw something that would exhibit symptoms of the influence of drugs.
7. Develop a study guide on a cassette for the major drug classifications.

Evaluation

Performance Objectives: The learner will:
1. Define the classification of drugs.
2. Understand the different effects of the various drugs.
3. Understand the difference between the use and abuse of drugs.
4. Know what common household substances are dangerous to the body.
5. Know the slang terms most often associated with drugs and drug use.

Addictive Behaviors

Drug Use Situations

BRUCE A. UHRICH *is a former instructor in the Health Education Division at the University of North Carolina at Greensboro. He is currently a graduate student in the Department of Health Education at Temple University, Philadelphia, Pennsylvania 19122.*

Under what conditions should the use of a drug be regarded as acceptable behavior in our society? To deal with this question I have developed, over the past two years, a series of statements which challenge student values and stimulate classroom discussion. I give students a handout with the following statements and these directions: "Read each statement carefully, then respond by rating each as an acceptable or unacceptable situation in which to use drugs. Be prepared to share each of your answers with the class, and to explain why you answered as you did."

Situation

1. Drinking an alcoholic beverage at a party.
2. Drinking an alcoholic beverage after work to relax at home.
3. Drinking an alcoholic beverage before driving several hundred miles.
4. Drinking an alcoholic beverage alone after an argument.
5. Drinking an alcoholic beverage at a football game.
6. Using a narcotic drug in a hospital for relief of pain following an operation.
7. Use of a narcotic drug by the head of a household in a lower socioeconomic area.
8. Use of a narcotic drug by a physician.
9. Use of a narcotic drug by students in an upper class high school.
10. Use of a narcotic drug as a cough suppressant.
11. Smoking tobacco in a high school restroom.
12. Smoking tobacco after dinner.
13. Smoking tobacco when meeting new people at a reception.
14. Smoking tobacco while riding in a car pool.
15. Smoking tobacco in class.
16. Using a sedative/tranquilizer to commit suicide.
17. Use of a sedative/tranquilizer to relax a neurotic personality.
18. Use of a sedative/tranquilizer to encourage sleep because of a loud roommate.
19. Use of a sedative/tranquilizer prescribed by a physician and then drinking heavily.
20. Use of a sedative/tranquilizer to relax before having to make a speech before a large group.
21. Utilizing marijuana at a dorm party.
22. Using marijuana after work to relax at home.
23. Refusing when handed a "joint" by your best friend.
24. Utilizing marijuana on a daily basis.
25. Using marijuana before an intramural softball game.
26. Starting each day with a cup of caffeine, before anything else.
27. Taking a "hit" of some stolen nitrous oxide.
28. Sniffing glue at a party.
29. Taking aspirin every time you feel any pain.
30. Receiving a painkilling drug from a paramedic for injuries at the scene of the accident.

Because the choices are limited to the extremes of acceptable or unacceptable, most students are highly motivated to verbally qualify their feelings. This situation allows the instructor to act as a true facilitator. For each statement, all students indicate by a show of hands which response they chose. Several students with acceptable and unacceptable ratings are then asked to explain their choice and supportive feelings. The result is class discussion, exposing all class members to a variety of opinions.

Chemically Dependent—
But Only for One Week

KATHLEEN FISCHER is a health teacher at the Orono Middle School, Long Lake, Minnesota. She is now in her second year of teaching and participated in the program described here last summer.

Hazelden (Center City, Minnesota), located 40 miles northeast of the Twin Cities, is a treatment center for chemically dependent people. This was the setting for an in-service education program for 80 educators this past summer. The program, in cooperation with the Minnesota Department of Education, was funded by a grant from the Hill Family Foundation. Eight educators per week were provided with a "live in" experience, participating in the full rehabilitation program with patients and staff. The purposes of the program were to develop a "gut level" feeling and attitude toward people with a dependency problem, to become more aware of the causes of chemical dependency problems, and to become aware that patients in treatment share the same basic needs with all men.

"God grant me the serenity to accept the things I cannot change, the courage to change the things I can, and the wisdom to know the difference." These words have taken on a much greater significance for me now after having spent a week at Hazelden. They are words which can be found in every room there, either inscribed on a wall plaque or being verbalized in group sessions. They are one part of the rehabilitation program for the chemically dependent person.[1] But what

---

[1] Chemically dependent refers here to a person who is dependent either on alcohol or drugs. Alcohol is also considered a drug, and it is considered to be the number one drug problem in this country.

does this have to do with rehabilitating chemically dependent people? During my "live in" experience I was able to grasp the impact of that simple verse and its meaning to the entire program, and despite the fact that I am not chemically dependent, my experience was realistic in every other sense.

Eight of us, four women and four men, came to Hazelden as patient-observers. Our backgrounds included public school teachers, high school counselors, and psychiatric clinic personnel. Each of us was assigned a different unit as our home for the week, which would be the essence of our experience. No two of us would have the same situation, and yet we all would have grappled with some intense feelings at the end of our stay.

Hazelden is in a picturesque setting. The long driveway has a way of quieting one's mind with a gentle peacefulness that all works for good here. A patient's first contact with the inside is the detoxification unit. Minimum stay in this area is at least one day, and most patients are eager to move to a unit as there is little to do here.

All of the treatment takes place in the units, which are essentially structured in a home-like atmosphere. There are three units for men and two for women. The only time all of the units are together is at meals and lectures, and then no fraternizing is allowed. The reason behind the no fraternization policy is to prevent patients from building up support groups which will set back their own rehabilitation. Our educator group, though, certainly appreciated the special afternoon sessions we had together. It was the first time I had found myself in an environment where I was the minority. And yet as the week progressed we discovered we were more alike than different.

Surprisingly enough, Hazelden is not harboring a group of skid row alcoholics. There is not a stereotype for a chemically dependent person. All of them are everyday real people—many of the women are housewives and mothers. There were young girls, quite a few older women, and two nuns there at that time. The number of older women surprised me, but it was pointed out that today is as good a day as any to start living a better life.

The day is rigidly scheduled for patients; this is to aid in their treatment, for at some point they must again start meeting these kinds of responsibilities. All three meals must be attended; each patient has a work responsibility such as vacuuming, cleaning the unit kitchen, etc.; morning, afternoon, and evening lectures must be attended; and daily group therapy sessions must be participated in. The rest of the day is spent reading assigned materials, meeting with staff, playing solitaire, sitting around the table drinking coffee and smoking cigarettes. (The cigarette consumption increases during a patient's stay at Hazelden. This could be expected since they are attempting to alleviate one problem at a time. The ever-present smoke, however, can be quite overwhelming to non-smokers.) No recreational pursuits are provided for patients. I found this confining for my usually independent nature, but the patient's purpose for being there is not for having a fun time.

The entire program is based on the Alcoholics Anonymous twelve steps. These steps basically require a person to surrender control of his life to a higher power (belief in God per se is not a requirement), to confess to oneself all one's faults and virtues, and to then confess this to another person. When a patient reaches the fifth step in the program he is then free to return to the outside world. The staff determines when a patient is ready to proceed to the next step, and this can be anxiety-producing for some patients who feel they are further along than the staff thinks.

Upon arrival at Hazelden, patients do not know how long they will be staying there. The normal period of time is approximately three to four weeks, although some patients may go into the extended care unit and remain up to a year. That unknowing fear can be a great stress factor in the rehabilitation. Most of them want to make their confinement as short as possible, but occasionally one will find a patient who has found Hazelden a secure place away from reality and would prefer to stay there. Few patients fully realize the personal depths to which their treatment will take them. Within them are the anxieties, frustrations, worries and resentments which carried them to the chemical escape they so desperately needed. Many of these people for the first time in their lives are having to face feelings they have hidden for years.

Each patient is treated according to his own personal needs. An essential part of recovery is learning to communicate feelings. Informal group therapy sessions aid in this task. In these sessions, patients are forced through questioning by the group to open up about themselves and get their true feelings out. The group can become quite hard on a person, and it is natural for people to avoid making responses that get at their feelings.

Patients do not have a magic formula prescribed for them when they leave so that they will not go back to chemicals. But if treatment has been effective they have much more than magic, for they have gained a self-understanding which can lead to a fuller, happier life. The stresses and difficulties of daily living are always present, and this is where their belief in a higher power must be strong.

The Hazelden experience is extremely worthwhile in a personal and professional sense. All of us should be given the opportunity to look within ourselves. All who are involved in the "helping" professions deal with people every day who are leading themselves to the brink where they only have one other out, and that may be chemicals. Each of us must take responsibility for sharing our own feelings and accepting these feelings as real. In turn, the process of self-acceptance can then go forth to others. This then will become the process we should use in preventing chemical dependency.

Our concern becomes that of the "feeling" life of people. Levi N. Larson, Education Director, North Dakota State Department of Health, says the real hope of drug abuse prevention lies in meeting the emotional needs of people—the need to be loved, to be heard, to be understood, the need to share feelings, the need to have meaningful communication with other people. Responding to these needs is how we get people off drugs. In doing this sooner lies the hope of keeping them from "getting on" drugs.

Addictive Behaviors

Learning by Teaching

ELAINE HALS is a teacher of health and physical education at South Shore High School in Brooklyn, New York. She is a new member of the SHR Editorial Board.

Drug education, an area of the health curriculum vital to high school students, is an area that easily turns young people off. They are tired of being preached to, moralized to, and lectured at. My dilemma was how to get the necessary information across, without losing the attention and interest of my health classes. I tried conventional lessons, contract teaching, and other methods, but somehow still lost them.

Last term I decided to let the students teach the unit to each other. I broke each of my classes into three committees and selected three of the most verbal members in each class to act as chairmen of the committees. The committees were selected by me so that there would be an equal number of verbal people in each group.

The three committees were:
1. Why drugs?
2. The facts.
3. Treatments available, including overdoses and emergency first aid.

In each class the committees had one day in class and two days in the library to organize their projects.

The committees had complete latitude in handling their subject, knowing that they had two days for their presentation. In one class for example "the why" committee spent one day on adults and drugs, and one day on young people and drugs. In the other class the committee dealt with drugs in advertising, sports, the school environment, and the home. In both classes the committee members asked questions of the class and involved them as part of the presentation. When it became necessary I was able to add information, ask questions, or guide the committee and the class. The students made up and ran off their own stencils, some brought in music of today that concerns itself with drugs, and one group even made up a role playing situation (and used class members to act it out).

The role playing situation was as follows: (a) parents waiting up for teenager to come home from party — young person comes home stoned; (b) reverse situation: teenage boy or girl waiting for parents to come home from a party—parents come home drunk.

This situation, and the discussion that followed, helped the students look at life for a moment from their parents' point of view, and to help them understand themselves in terms of their tolerance for others. The students listened to each other

and were nonjudgmental. No value judgments were made, but the information necessary for the students to make their own value judgments and their own decisions was available. This information was given to them by a source that they were willing to listen to—their classmates.

It was a worthwhile experience for the class, and for me. The students in my classes felt free to express their opinions as well as their knowledge. They had a chance to step into the teacher's role for a short while and to see the class from a different point of view. The students received not only the needed information of the drug unit but experience in working in a group and seeing their project through to completion. The unit was more meaningful than if I had taught it.

After evaluation, the students found some flaws: (a) people came unprepared to give their reports and (b) people read long technical reports not meaningful to the class. In general, they favored this method. As for me, I really got to hear about and understand the drug "problem" from a young people's point of view.

This is an approach that I will use again.

Aging: A Need for Sensitivity

KENNETH A. BRIGGS is an assistant professor of health education at the State University of New York, College at Cortland, Cortland, New York 13045.

With our culture's shift from revering the old to worshipping youth and the breakdown of the extended family into separate nuclear units which usually exclude the elderly, a whole generation of young people are uneducated and insensitive to the elderly and their needs. Comprehensive school health education, which seeks to improve the quality of life through informed choices, is a good place to educate school age children about aging. It not only makes students more aware and sensitive to the needs of the elderly; it also educates them for their own aging.

Following are some suggestions to help create an awareness and caring for the elderly and their problems. These exercises help show students what it is like to be old in a culture that treats senior citizens the way we do.

Sensory Deprivation Simulation Exercises

The following simulation exercises try to bring to the young and healthy a sensitivity to what it must be like to be old and suffering from common sensory insults reported by the elderly.

Arthritis (reported by 33 out of 100 elderly)

Using cellophane tape, tape students' fingers together in various combinations, e.g., tape thumb and index finger together and the 4th and 5th fingers together. Wrap elastic bandages around the knees to simulate stiff knees. Have students perform simple tasks and then share their experiences of what it might be like to be old and have arthritis.

Visual Handicaps (reported by 15 out of 100 elderly)

Take sunglasses or laboratory protective glasses and smear vaseline on them until you get your desired visual loss. Have students wear the glasses and perform everyday things such as reading a

menu or a newspaper, or look up the phone number of a pharmacy that will deliver prescriptions to old people (if there is one). Have students record and share their reactions.

Hearing Loss (reported by 22 out of 100 elderly)

Place a cotton ball in the student's exterior ear canal. For a more pronounced effect, have them also wear headphones or earmuffs. Have students listen to the TV or radio at a low level, or try to carry on a conversation with someone who has no hearing loss and must shout at them to be heard. Again, have students share their feelings.

Loss of Touch

Cover the students' fingers with rubber cement and after it dries, have them try to thread a needle.

Loss of Smell

Have students taste various foods while pinching their nostrils shut.

Multiplicity (polymorbidity)

Certainly many elderly people suffer from many aging insults. They may have a hearing loss, arthritis, and a visual handicap. To help students understand multiplicity and what it might be like, have several students perform tasks with various combinations of the above simulations. For example, one student can simulate finger arthritis, visual loss, and loss of touch and smell then go to the cafeteria and buy a carton of milk. Upon returning, have the stu-

dent share some of his feelings during the experience as an older person with sensory deprivation. Be sure to exercise necessary safety precautions when students perform such simulations.

Songs and the Elderly

A lot of popular songs have been written recently that do a good job of developing a caring sensitivity and awareness of the elderly in listeners. Following are some examples of such songs and their artists.

"Old Man"—Neil Young
"Old Friends" "Voices of Old People"—Simon and Garfunkel
"When I'm Sixty-Four" "Eleanor Rigby"—The Beatles
"Two Lonely Old People"—Wings
"Hello Old Friend"—Eric Clapton
"Lonely People"—America
"Good Company"—Queen
"Hello in There"—Bette Midler
"I Never Thought I'd Live to be 100" "Travelin' Eternity Road"—Moody Blues
"Let Time Go Lightly"—Harry Chapin
"Father and Son" "But I Might Die Tonight"—Cat Stevens

A nice touch to make aging education come alive in the classroom is to add slides of old people to the music. It can be quite powerful in creating sensitivity to aging.

Activities for Application and Discussion

Have students share some of their fears about growing old.

Have students draw pictures of themselves showing what they will be like when they are 100 years old. What losses do they show?

Have students think of or photograph things in a grocery store that demonstrate our insensitivity to the aged such as, unit pricing numbers and prices that are too small to read, bulk packaging, no carry out service.

Have someone in class carry on a conversation with another person in class who has simulated speech problems that follow a stroke by placing a ping pong ball in his/her mouth.

Use the following opinionnaire to generate discussion about the elderly.

Indicate to the right of each statement whether you agree or disagree.

1. Old people are better off living with other old people.
2. Old people need rehabilitation.
3. Rehabilitation is done best in a nursing home.
4. Sixty-five is a good age at which to retire.
5. Old people live happier lives away from the young, competitive world.
6. Old people should be kept active.
7. Old people suffer a sense of loss when their children leave home.
8. Our society encourages old people to be productive and useful.
9. Old people should stay in their own homes, if possible.
10. Old people should be discouraged from dependent relationships with agency personnel.
11. Most older people are ready to rest and don't want to be involved in "doing things."
12. Old people cannot learn as well as young people because of deterioration of the brain associated with aging.

There are two films that are a must to use when trying to create a caring sensitivity of the aged in our young people:

Trigger Films on Aging —This is an excellent film dramatizing five brief situations common to the elderly. The film is excellent in eliciting emotions and a free flow of thoughtful discussion from its viewers. Produced by the University of Michigan Television Center, 400 South 4th St., Ann Arbor, MI 48103.

Peege—A marvelously produced, emotionally charged film of a young man who is successful where others failed in breaking down the communication barrier between his aged grandmother and a family who doesn't understand her. Distributed by Phoenix Films, 470 Park Ave. South, New York, NY 10016.

Take two pictures of, for example, a street corner or the entrance steps to a bus. One picture of your chosen scene should be in focus and the other should purposely be out of focus. This will dramatically demonstrate the problems encountered by those elderly who have a serious vision loss and the insensitivity we have to these people by having such things as "Do Not Walk" signs that are too small to read.

We cannot overlook the most obvious and valuable resource of all—the elderly themselves. Bring the elderly to the students or take the students to the elderly. Allow them to ask questions of each other, spend time together, and most important of all, try to understand each other.

Because of the nature of our modern society and quite often the insensitivity it carries with it for the elderly, health education about and for aging that tries to reintroduce the elderly to those who may be out of touch and insensitive to them is imperative. Such education can be valuable for the aged as well for all those who may better understand the exigencies of the years to come.

Aging

Picnic in the Park
Humanizing an Aging Unit in a Personal Health Class

MICHAEL J. GAETA is a doctoral candidate and graduate teaching assistant in the Department of Health Education, Oregon State University, Corvallis, Oregon 97330.

Students in my Personal Health class had a picnic in the park with 54 elderly residents from Heart of the Valley Retirement Center and Nursing Home Complex in Corvallis, Oregon as the culmination of a unit on aging. In planning the aging unit I decided to design a program that would provide the students with an accurate knowledge base of the biological, psychological, and sociological aspects of aging; and even more important, provide them with experiences that would sensitize them to the realities of aging. All of this was to be terminated in a picnic, a celebration of life bringing the young together with the old.

"Ageism" is prejudice and discrimination leveled by one age group against another.[1] It is just as volatile and injust as other forms of bigotry such as racism and sexism. It is founded upon ignorance, myth, stereotypes, and fear. It results in alienation, despair, deprivation, powerlessness, and even hostility. The only way to combat this prejudice is to meet it head on with accurate information and experiences that will demonstrate to people of all ages how cruel it is to think of our elders as inhuman.

A total of six class periods were devoted to the aging unit. We started the first class with Palmore's "Facts on Aging" quiz,[2] which covers basic facts and misconceptions about aging. The quiz takes approximately 10 minutes to administer, but stimulates much discussion about basic physical, mental, and social facts and the most frequent misconceptions about aging. The quiz contains factual information documented by empirical data. This tool is an excellent resource that provides the students with a relevant vehicle for more clearly understanding the multidimensional topic of aging.

The second class was devoted to a cursory examination of the more common and current biological theories of aging. The primary objective was to familiarize the students with the present theory of the etiology of senescence. An excellent comprehensive review of the biological theories of aging is found in the *Handbook of the Biology of Aging*. It provides an excellent framework.[3]

In the third class session students had the opportunity to discuss aging with a 69-year-old senior activist. Several days before the class students were instructed to write down any questions they had about any aspect of aging. The guest speaker was given the questions a few days ahead of her scheduled talk so that she could more accurately ascertain the needs and concerns of the students.

Sitting in a large circle with the class, the speaker answered questions and related her philosophy of life so eloquently that the entire class was caught up in her bubbling enthusiasm for life. She shared her feelings on everything from sexuality to death. After a standing ovation, the students without coercion lined up and one by one proceeded to hug and kiss her as they left the class. It was obvious that those students went away with a more positive and beautiful perspective on aging.

The fourth class period consisted of aging simulation games. With the help and expertise of a gerontology professor, the students were divided into groups of five. Shoe boxes filled with paraphernalia to simulate impairments brought on by the aging process were passed out to each group. Arthritic, visual, hearing, aphasic, and stroke impairments were simulated as part of the exercise. Each "impaired individual" was given a task to do alone. This was followed up by a group task. These simulations enabled the students to more realistically understand the impairments and restrictions that many aged people live with each day. For an excellent review of aging simulation games see *Health Education* September/October 1977.[4]

In class five a gerontological counselor addressed the area of psychosocial needs of the elderly. The counselor emphasized that we are all creatures of need—to be fed, kept warm and dry, to grow and develop at our own pace, to be held, caressed, recognized, loved and stimulated. While most people recognize the importance of practicing and subscribing to these tenets in the early years of human development, many of us forget that these needs must be met from cradle to grave if we are to reach

**Gazette-Times Photos
By Tom Warren**

Laurence Garner, left, talks with student Mark Rabichaud.

Lunch in the park

The 40 students in Michael Gaeta's Personal Health class at Oregon State had a special final examination—a box lunch in Chintimini Park with 40 residents of Heart of the Valley Center.

Jeanette Stoner, Rosemary Wick, Barbara Quinn and Cindy Miller entertained by singing to the senior citizens.

Jeannette, who is a freshman pre-veterinarian student from Hood River, said students brought their own lunches and exchanged them with a senior.

"It was the neatest final I've ever taken," she said. "I used to be afraid of growing old, but I learned from the seniors that they have a lot of fun, have hobbies and really get around the community." She said she's also learned how they cope with arthritis, hearing and seeing problems.

On Friday, June 2 1978, the **Gazette-Times** of Corvallis, Oregon ran this picture story about the class described by Gaeta in this article. The photographs on this page were taken by Tom Warren.

Youngsters and oldsters soak up the sunshine.

Danita Ruzic, chats with Cora Warner, holding cup, at the picnic in Chintimini Park. Danita has been spending each morning at Heart of the Valley Center and produced a term paper on her experiences.

Kimberly Koehler, left, helps Marian Taylor with her picnic lunch.

78

optimum growth and development. This last session put the finishing touches on preparing the students for the picnic with the elderly.

Working in conjunction with the activities director from Heart of the Valley Retirement Center and Nursing Home the groundwork was laid for the picnic. The picnic called for the exchange of box lunches with the elderly. The students were asked to prepare a lunch complete with treats not usually found in an institution. Arrangements were made through the administrator for the Center cafeteria to provide box lunches for the students plus lemonade and coffee for the entire group.

The activities director took care of publicizing the event at the Center. Signs were placed in the elevator and on the bulletin boards notifying the residents of the picnic. A list of potential participants from the nursing section was compiled and these patients were contacted and asked if they would like to attend the event.

The park chosen for the picnic was one block away from the Center so no bus transportation was necessary. However, since our group would have to cross a busy street to get to the park, the Corvallis police were contacted and they agreed to provide traffic direction and assistance.

The local newspaper was contacted and told of the picnic in the park. It was thought that the publicity would be good for both the Heart of the Valley Center and the health education department.

The day of the picnic was beautiful. The sky was blue, the sun was shining and the temperature was pleasant. I arrived at the Center at 11:30 and found patients lined up in the lobby eagerly waiting to depart. The police arrived shortly thereafter and were given instructions as to when we would depart and what route we would traverse to reach the park. Within a matter of minutes students started to arrive and we began hooking them up with residents from the Center. As I looked out of the main doors, the group of elders and students reminded me of a beautiful parade. A meeting of the young and the old. People with canes, some in wheelchairs, all being escorted by students. Human beings that had been separated by walls, not walls of wood or stone, but walls of ignorance and fear, were sharing love, food, talk, and companionship. As I moved about the group taking pictures, I was amazed at the rate and quality of interaction that was happening all around me.

Students with musical talents played harmonica, guitar and sang to entertain the group. Song sheets of old time favorites printed in large block type were distributed and the whole group joined in the merriment by singing songs, clapping hands, tapping feet, and laughing.

After sharing lunch in the warm sun, gifts were handed out to the elderly by the students. With the extra gifts students suggested that we have a contest and hand out gifts in descending order from oldest to youngest. A 94-year-old grandmother won first prize.

Time seemed to fly by and before we knew it the time had come to leave the park. On the way back to the Center traffic was blocked up both ways on Harrison Boulevard, as students and residents moved in a procession that stretched from the park to the Center. Residents and staff from the Center were in the windows waving to our group as we arrived.

The reactions from students and elders alike was unequivocally positive. No sooner did we get back to the Center than one elderly woman asked when the next picnic was to be scheduled.

Without any question, it was obvious that many of the fears, myths, and stereotypes of aging were bashed down that day. With a little bit of imagination, coordination, planning, and cooperation, a picnic in the park on a sunny day in May gave a group of personal health students the opportunity to learn first hand that aging is not all negative and that old people are no different from young people.

[1]Butler, Robert N. "Ageism: Another Form of Bigotry." Gerontologist, 1969, Vol. 9: 243–46.

[2]Palmore, Erdman. "Facts on Aging—A Short Quiz." Gerontologist, 1977, Vol. 17, No 4.: pp. 315–20.

[3]Finch, Caleb E. and Leonard Hayflide (eds.) Handbook of the Biology of Aging, Van Nostrand Reinhold Co., New York, 1977.

[4]Briggs, Kenneth. "Aging: A Need for Sensitivity." Health Education, Sept./Oct. 1977, pp. 37–38.

HEALTH ANAGRAMS

KATHLEEN M. SIEGWARTH is instructor, Department of Health and Physical Education, Bowling Green State University, Bowling Green, Ohio 43403.

Health educators realize that the techniques used in teaching can serve as catalysts to the material being presented. One way to help students learn about health care specialists in the community health unit of the health education curriculum is with anagrams. The procedure consists of using handouts containing anagrams, which when properly unscrambled spell out occupations in the health care profession. They are constructed to read as names. Under the caption "My Name Is" the anagrams are listed in columns and opposite is a column headed by "My Occupation Is" with appropriate blanks. Periods are not to be considered in translation, but all letters must be used.

Example:

My Name Is	My Occupation Is
1. Stu Coil	1. _____

The correct answer is oculist.

Here are several ways this idea might be used in class.

1. Distribute the sheet one week prior to the scheduled lesson day. Make it an individual contest whereby the student with the most correct answers would receive recognition as determined by the teacher. In case of a tie, a "playoff" would be held in class. New words would be put forth and a time limit set. When time expires the one with the most correct answers is the winner. Have the other students work the same problems. They then can offer any answers missed by the contestants and rate their own accomplishment.

2. Divide the class into two teams. Have each group elect a captain who is responsible for recording the solution for each anagram and serves as their spokesman. Allow 30 minutes for each team to work. Validate the answers between the two teams at the end of the time limit. The team with the most correct answers is the winner. Should a tie occur a playoff is held immediately, with a five minute time limit.

3. Group anagrams into similar categories. For example, psychiatrist, psy-

chologist, and analyst. This enables the teacher to distribute them during the unit in which they are pertinent.

4. Release the anagrams in groups of five or ten daily over a one to two week period. Answers to the problems may be turned in the next day and new ones distributed. A winner is declared after all answers have been submitted.

Following is a list of 45 anagrams with the appropriate answers.

	My Name Is	My Occupation Is
1.	Heston Satisgole	Anesthesiologist
2.	Les G. Trail	Allergist
3.	Lenore Vut	Volunteer
4.	Sandie Sure	Nurse's Aide
5.	Togol I. Scadir	Cardiologist
6.	Hope Toast	Osteopath
7.	Lori N. Stouge	Neurologist
8.	Tobias T. Nicer	Obstetrician
9.	Phil O. Mostogoth	Ophthomologist
10.	Patti Goolsh	Pathologist
11.	Nate I. Picidar	Pediatrician
12.	Chris T. Stipay	Psychiatrist
13.	Sol Goitur	Urologist
14.	Gail T. Sodoir	Radiologist
15.	Gib O. Loist	Biologist
16.	Tania M. Torrids	Administrator
17.	Tad I. Porsit	Podiatrist
18.	Seth Doorpit	Orthopedist
19.	G. O. Nurse	Surgeon
20.	Rod Ryle	Orderly
21.	Ted Tins	Dentist
22.	Thor Stondoit	Orthodontist
23.	Ricator Porch	Chiropractor
24.	Gipsy T. School	Psychologist
25.	T. S. Chime	Chemist
26.	Tod Roc	Doctor
27.	Unis T. Tortini	Nutritionist
28.	Patricia Pylsthesh	Physical Therapist
29.	Nyle G. Gostico	Gynecologist
30.	Thom Toilgoes	Hemotologist
31.	Scott Goily	Cytologist
32.	Nat I. Eidic	Dietician
33.	Stanlie Chet Comlodig	Medical Technologist
34.	Caine Y. Xanchirt	X-ray Technician
35.	Peter Lance Grantitoir	General Practitioner
36.	Toni Priceset	Receptionist
37.	Mort G. Sealdito	Dermatologist
38.	Mic A. Prade	Paramedic
39.	Sy A. Lant	Analyst
40.	I. N. Rent	Intern
41.	I. C. Shypain	Physician
42.	R. E. Sun	Nurse
43.	Pam C. H. Stair	Pharmacist
44.	Morie T. Topst	Optometrist
45.	Cher E. Raser	Researcher

Consumer Wellness, One School's Approach

JON W. HISGEN is a health instructor in Pewaukee Public Schools, 210 Main Street, Pewaukee, Wisconsin 53072 and an instructor of consumer health for the University of Wisconsin, Milwaukee.

Every year I instruct my consumer health units at the seventh and ninth grade levels I am made acutely aware of people's trusting nature. In this "credit card culture" where we exist, instant pleasures are a signature away. There is no better example of this approach to consumer decisions than in the world of health products and services. We blindly use hit or miss tactics in everything from wiping out those unsightly blemishes with steam to strengthening our rectus abdominus muscle with electric belts.

The condition of wellness is a combination of many interacting forces, including the individuals' environment, their reaction to it, associations, psychological background, and ability to accept attitudinal change. Today's health consumer is more likely to face these forces after his/her health has been threatened in some way. Consumer wellness is not an easily acquired status but must be learned.

My initial seventh grade consumer health activity is to sell each student a bottle of Dr. Lemke's Stomachic Drops using a stereotypical medicine man approach. The following is an example of the pitch I use to convince the class the product works.

1. I tell students about a college assignment to recreate a medicine from an old medical text.
2. I chose Dr. Lemke's drops because of its advertised ability to cure both acne problems and split ends (7th grade concerns).
3. The mysterious ingredient is capsicum that must be imported from Africa and grown hydroponically.
4. I finished making the product in two months and successfully field tested it on my friends and myself.
5. I unsuccessfully asked for support from the AMA and Bristol Meyers.
6. I decided to market the product through magazines after receiving a patent on the product.
7. I bought a factory to grow capsicum and produce Dr. Lemke's drops.

8. Sales have increased each year for the last three years.
9. Famous people have endorsed the product (the Osmonds, the Jackson Five).
10. A local newspaper is coming to take advertising pictures of students holding the product.
11. If the students bring the money next time we meet, I'll give them a special offer of two bottles for the price of one.

Over the past five years around 91% of the students have agreed to bring the cost of the product the next day while in fact 70% actually did. When I tell the students that a cruel hoax was played upon them the following responses can be heard: "I'll never trust you again." "We thought you were above that." "Well, you certainly made me look foolish." "I was just playing along with your little game."

The alarmingly high number of gullible consumers pointed out the need for

some direction in our consumer health program. Out of this we instituted a consumer health program entitled WISE MAN.

W ise
I independent   M otivate
S afe/effective A ware
E valuate   N otable

Each of the letters represented a competency we wanted our students to have by the time they left our health program.
1. The student will be able to make *wise* and careful decisions about the consumer products and services he/she uses (consumer health protection).
2. The student will be able to make decisions *independent* of outside influences (e.g. advertising, pseudo-science, etc.).
3. The student will be able to choose products and services that are both *safe* and *effective*.

Photos by Jon W. Hisgen

4. The student will be able to *evaluate* new and existing health products and services (the work of government agencies, insurance programs, alternative medical practices, etc.).
5. The students will be able to *motivate* others in their present or future family to make wise consumer health decisions (well-thought out family medicine chests and first aid kits).
6. The student will be *aware* of pitfalls facing the consumer of health products and services (quackery, superstitions, fads, and fallacies).
7. The students will be able to make *notable* savings in their consumer health budget and notable improvement in their overall wellness.

Our school's consumer health program is based on these competencies. A copy of our consumer health curriculum and methods guide can be obtained by writing the author.

A Healthy Consumer Health Class

TOM McFARLAND is a consumer education specialist at the Family Life Education Center, Toledo Public Schools, Toledo, Ohio 43604. ANN RUDRAUFF is educative services specialist for WGTE-TV, Channel 30, in Toledo.

Our experience has shown that the most successful way to teach consumer health is to throw out traditional classes and have students learn by doing, using the community as a classroom. Most of the learning experiences we describe are oriented toward high school or college level but adaptations can be made to suit various school aged or community groups.

Advertising

Thorough understanding of how advertising works is necessary for the consumer health student. Some suggested activities are:

Ad substantiation campaign. Survey local media for advertisements of health and beauty products. Printed ads can be brought to class; radio and TV ads can be taped for discussion. Many ad agencies and TV and radio stations throw away their tapes and layouts and are happy to see someone get some use from them.

Claims made in the ads are scrutinized and some are selected for analysis. Students write company presidents and ask for factual substantiation of the advertisement. This is examined to see if the claim is justified. The information gathered can be shared with classmates and can be made public.

Counter-ads. Since advertising is obviously biased, consumers deserve to hear the other side of the story. Students prepare counter-ads such as, "aspirin is all the same, it may cause internal bleeding." A visit to an ad agency or asking an advertising man in as guest instructor can help students prepare their ads. Students should then try to get local media to use their counter-ads as public service spots.

Fraudulent charities. Most of the fraudulent groups are centered around research in disease prevention and cure, and they have bilked consumers out of millions of dollars. In this project to ex-

pose such operations, students paint and label empty coffee cans with "American Cancer Center," "National School for Epileptics" or some other phony health agency name. Working in pairs, the students take money and write down pledges. After counting the money, it is returned to donors with an explanation. This activity should be widely publicized so that they can learn without being unnecessarily embarrassed. More people will know they should check before giving.

Health Insurance

Health insurance is a crucial issue about which few consumers have a working knowledge. One way to identify and probe health insurance issues is by values clarification techniques.

Voting on pertinent questions. How many of you have health insurance? How many are covered under a family policy? How many are covered under a group policy? How many have Blue Cross-Blue Shield? How many can list the exclusions in their policy?

Forced choice questions. These help students decide which alternative they prefer: private medicine or socialized medicine; unnecessary luxury or necessity? Students can vote by moving to either side of the room, then find someone there to discuss the reasons for their decision. The teacher can design questions to bring out important points to be discussed.

Values continuums. Use to encourage participation in discussion of current issues related to health insurance. Health costs are: too high—just right—too low. Medicine should be: socialized—totally private. Health insurance is: a waste—all right—crucial. I usually block out the center of the continuum to discourage students who find it too easy to be indifferent.

Rank order. (1) List major exclusions found in insurance policies. Rank in order of danger to consumers. (2) List ways to learn about health insurance and rank in order of preference. Teachers can use this list in planning classes. (3) List types of health insurance coverage, and rank in order of importance to the consumer or in order of expense, such as: basic hospital, major medical, dental rider, maternity benefits. Students can share their rationales for rankings in groups of three.

Price Comparison Research

These research results can shed much light on future buying practices. A certain type of product is selected for study by

groups of students. Types of health products good for study include: prescription drugs, over-the-counter drugs, perishable foods, cosmetics, or food sold in a health food store.

After groups are formed, students plan to visit a variety of stores such as a chain food store, small pharmacy, and discount store. Prices may vary depending on location of the store, so encourage students to visit suburban, rural, and urban areas, if possible. Items to be price-checked should be standardized by brand, size, weight, count, or whatever, so results will be comparable and accurate.

Groups can make charts to depict their results, analysis of data, and conclusions. Presentations to the whole class should be made.

Health Practitioner Interviews

The teacher can assign job classifications or let students select the one they are most interested in, to go out and interview someone in that area. Several possible candidates are listed under "guest speaker" later in the article.

Make sure students are aware of how to contact people, set up interviews, and ask pertinent, interesting questions. Role playing in the classroom before the interview will give confidence to carry out the project successfully.

Follow up activities include: oral reports, role play, group comparisons of categories, mock debates with students playing the role of the person interviewed, and so on.

General

Guest speakers. A wealth of information can be provided to students by outside experts. This is especially helpful if field trips are not within the budget. Teachers can call on a wide selection of community people including:

Health practitioners—doctors, pharmacists, paramedics, nurses, public health officials, nutritionists.

Governmental or voluntary agencies—Better Business Bureau, Consumer Protection Agency, Post Office, local health departments, civic groups.

Educators—university health staff, consumer specialists, other teachers from the school.

Business—insurance agents, food packers, advertising agencies, credit bureaus, health food store owners, cosmetologists, lawyers.

If a speaker's time is limited, tape the presentation for the rest of the classes. Invite several guest speakers at once to form a panel or have a debate on a given topic. Preparing the speakers and students ahead of time and following up makes this more effective.

Pretest. This is a good way to assess the group's knowledge, misconceptions, background, values, and behavior. It can be used to learn what the students want to know or as a springboard for discussion. If the test includes content-based information covering the entire course, it can be used as a posttest.

Some sample questions are:

1. Content-based items (true or false)— Toothpastes are necessary for good dental health; the best relief of arthritis pain is prescription drugs; gargles or mouthwashes are not effective treatment for sore throats. 2. Attitude and behavior-based items—I see a doctor and a dentist at least once a year; I am adequately covered by medical insurance; I have a good credit rating. 3. Unfinished sentences—I spend money foolishly on_____; I really shop around for _____.

Experiment with some of the activities described here; adapt and apply them to your own teaching situation. Remember, an involved class is a "healthy" class.

Consumer Health

The Teenage Consumer

LEE ANN LARSON is a 7th and 8th grade health teacher at the Dexter McCarty Middle School, Gresham, Oregon.

The marketplace is wide open to today's teenage consumer. As the target of constant bombardment by advertisers, the teenager with access to money is in the position of making decisions with very little information. Health products, in particular, appeal to the teenager with their promises to beautify. Although information for the student in this vital area is hard to find, I teach a unit with seventh and eighth graders to develop awareness of consumer health education.

To understand any new body of knowledge familiarity with the terms that relate to that area is necessary. The students' first task is to find definitions of appropriate words. We use health books rather than dictionaries to give students specific subject definitions rather than general definitions which they may have trouble applying to topical situations. This list of words introduces the unit:

bait and switch	media
code-dating system	nostrum
comparison shopping	patent medicine
consumer	product
cosmetic	proprietary compound
dentifrice	quack
fraud	trademark
indirect lie	

The students next investigate some facts about their role as consumers. What is the history of health products and services? What about the "medicine man" of the old west and his cure-all drugs? How are his claims different from or the same as advertising that we might hear or see today? Students investigate how advertising affects the consumer and just how much advertising is directed at their age group and why. They take a look at how Americans spend their health dollar, and of total income how many of their dollars are spent for health products and services.

Middle-school students are still secure with the thought that if they get sick or hurt their parents or some other adult will make sure they are taken care of properly. This unit's lessons present them with situations and factual histories in which they must make some decisions of their own. What if their doctor tells them that they have a disease which cannot be cured, but they read about a doctor who can cure the disease? What if they are told they have cancer of the leg and it must be amputated, but someone knows of a doctor who has a cure for cancer? The possibilities are endless and the

cases do not even have to be so dramatic. This leads to an investigation of quackery and a realization that they are one of the prime target groups because of their susceptibility. Mail-order quackery traps them with its glamour and seeming privacy of the postal system. They get involved with researching training, signs, and results of quackery.

Students can become pretty outraged about what quacks are "getting away with." At this point, students investigate some of the organizations working in some way to protect the consumer from fraud. They study the Food and Drug Administration, Federal Trade Commission, U.S. Postal Service, American Medical Association, Consumer's Union, and Better Business Bureau. Throughout the discussions, students are reminded that these organizations are handicapped by their dependence on consumer complaints to act. If the consumer is too ashamed, too afraid, or too lazy to report an incident or complaint, other unsuspecting consumers will be subjected to the same treatment by a fraudulant person or company.

Even if students have some information on quacks and the groups which protect the consumer, they are still left with the problem of what to look for in good medical services. Investigation continues with some of the guidelines to follow in selecting a physician followed by a review of specialists (pediatrician, general practitioner, internist, surgeon, psychiatrist, etc.). Students need to look for the physician best able to handle their needs at various stages in life. An increasingly important aspect of medical service is that provided by hospitals. Students try to find out what kinds of hospitals exist and what questions should be answered before choosing a hospital.

The next project gets students involved in investigating a product. With school funds, I purchased three brands of several products from a discount store, adding another price to the label from a regular grocery store or drug store. The products used were aspirin, toothpaste, shampoo, deodorant, vitamin tablets, ready-to-eat cereal, and acne preparations. Knowing seventh and eighth grade students, I emptied all of the containers before using them in the classroom. The class arranged itself in groups to provide an equal number to work on each product. To make it somewhat fair, each group drew a number to indicate its turn at choosing a product. Once the preliminaries were settled, each group received a form on which to write the information to present to the class. The questions include:

1. What is the history of the product? (Where did it come from? Who found it and how? How long has it been around?)

2. What are the ingredients as they are listed on the label of the product?

3. What are the uses for the product as listed on the label?

4. Can this product cause any harm? (Not only the particular brands they are investigating, but any other brand of the same product. In most cases this information is not on the label so they will have to do further reading.)

5. Is any brand of this product better than others? Where did you find that information? (Students have a tendency to rely on advertising, written or word-of-mouth, to make this decision. Encourage them to use resource materials to see if they can find reliable information.)

6. What is the price comparison for the product? (Comparing the same brand at two different stores, different brands at the same store, and different sizes of the same brand. I purchased the products, as much as possible in the same size, but students sometimes take it upon themselves to check on other sizes.)

7. What is the latest information about this product? (I collected all the information I could—magazine and newspaper articles—about a product and let the students decide what is significant enough to report to the rest of the class.)

8. What do advertisements for this product look or sound like? (Students can cut ads from magazines to show or report ones they have heard on the radio or from friends, or seen on television.)

The reports to the class can produce more questions and further research plus a wealth of basic information.

One of the common concerns to come from this investigation is the inadequate information found on the labeling standards and new ones currently under consideration. Included in the unit are not only the products investigated, but any product which may in some way relate to health and safety, such as baby cribs and toys. This is also an excellent time to get into nutrition labeling. A fun exercise is for students to design a label for a product, including all of the information they think is important for the consumer.

Another way to get students thinking about health products and selections is to have them collect advertisements about many different brands of some product.

After students decide which brand of the product is best, using only the advertisements, each will tell how confident he feels in his decision. The students will also indicate other information they would like to have to make an even better choice.

Sources of Information

Information in this particular area can be difficult to find. Some of the sources found to be useful include:

Books

Editors of Consumer Reports. *The Medicine Show.* New York: Consumers Union, 1971.

Jones, Kenneth L. and others. *Consumer Health.* San Francisco: Canfield Press, 1971.

Kime, Robert E. *Health: A Consumers Dilemma.* Belmont, California: Wadsworth Publishing Company, Inc., 1970.

Richmond, Juilus B., M.D. *Health and Growth.* Book 7 and book 8. Glenview, Illinois: Scott, Foresman and Company, 1972.

Magazines

Consumer Reports
Today's Health

Bulletins and Pamphlets

Facts on Quacks—What You Should Know About Health Quackery. Chicago: American Medical Association, 1971.

Fads, Myths, Quacks—and Your Health. Public Affairs Pamphlet No. 415. New York: Public Affairs Committee, Inc., 1972.

Health Quackery: Devices. Chicago: American Medical Association, 1968.

Medicines Your Doctor Prescribes. Washington, D.C.: Pharmaceutical Manufacturers Association.

People and the City—Buyers Beware. Glenview, Illinois: Scott, Foresman and Company, 1972.

Responsible Consumer, The. Public Affairs Pamphlet No. 453. New York: Public Affairs Committee, Inc., 1970.

We Want You To Know About F.D.A. Food and Drug Administration Publication No. 1. Rockville, Maryland: Food and Drug Administration.

Crisis Hot Line Experience

ALOYSIUS J. JANGL is health education instructor and subject area coordinator at Ardsley Middle School, Ardsley, New York 10502.

The emergence and impact of two relatively new mental health concerns, death and suicide education, can be viewed as outgrowths of the education system attempting to ensure healthy personality development. Nevertheless, mental health areas within the health education curriculum are often neglected or poorly presented. Why? Perhaps the curriculum is largely fact-oriented with little accommodation for the bulk of affective content involved in mental health. The wealth of emotions and attitudes combined with inexperience and/or fear of affective teaching may make some health educators apprehensive about such vital health areas.

With statistics climbing, suicide is now the third leading cause of death among young people between the ages of 15 and 19, and it ranks first or second on college campuses. The area of suicide and its prevention should be of vital concern to the health educator. Suicidology, the scientific study of suicide, investigates the many complex causes leading individuals to self-destructive behavior. Research has shown that suicides are not spontaneous. There are clues that foreshadow this behavior to which both educator and student alike can become sensitized. Armed with this awareness and sensitivity, preventive and reinforcing steps can be taken to help the individual. It is erroneous to assume that handling suicidal behavior or any "abnormal" behavior is the psychiatrist's or psychologist's province alone. Suicide prevention is not exclusively a medical or psychiatric problem. Health educators can operate within certain limits in teaching and counseling. Moreover, they can help shoulder their mental health responsibility by presenting the essential facts concerning crisis behavior in a meaningful way to their students.

The following is an example of an instructional strategy that has been used in a middle school mental health unit dealing with crisis prevention and intervention. It may encourage other health educators toward more effective affective teaching and the rewarding experience of humanistic health education.

Behavioral Objectives for Students

1. Cite particular situations which have the potential for critical or self-destructive behavior.

2. Devise a reference list of persons, groups, or agencies that deal with suicide or attempted suicide.
3. Identify clues in the individual's behavior that suggest a need for consultation with a professional specialist or a need for other forms of immediate help.
4. Identify and suggest various constructive alternatives and psychological first aid advice.

Instructional Materials

1. Battery operated walkie-talkie; 50 ft. extension.
2. Record player with microphone and speaker jacks; speaker with 50 ft. extension jack cord; microphone jack cord.
3. Thirty or more dittos of Crisis Hot Line Evaluation Sheet.

CRISIS HOT LINE EVALUATION SHEET

Instructions
Place the name of the student who is the crisis hot line operator in the numbered box atop each column. While listening carefully to the conversation, check off, in the vertical column under each operator's name, the psychological first aid advice he suggests.

PSYCHOLOGICAL First Aid	NAME OF OPERATOR				
	1.	2.	3.	4.	5.
Listens attentively					
Takes complaints seriously					
Evaluates seriousness of intention					
Examines intensity of emotional disturbance					
Assesses resources available					
Does something tangible					
Affirmative, yet supportive					
Asks directly about suicidal thoughts and intent					
Not misled by passing second thoughts					
Suggests personal or professional assistance					

This evaluation sheet has been formulated from the article "Ecological Aspects of Self-Destruction: Some Legal, Legislative and Behavioral Implications," by Calvin Frederick in *Health and Human Values* by Allure Jefcoat (John Wiley & Sons, Inc., New York, 1972) pp. 172-80.

Instructional Activity

Instruct each student in the class to write out a critical situation which would warrant a call to a local crisis hot line center. Next, distribute a Crisis Hot Line Evaluation Sheet to each student. Select one student who wishes to be the crisis hot line caller and another student to be the crisis hot line operator. The hot line caller will be stationed outside the classroom speaking into the microphone, thus relating the incident to the entire class within the room via the extension speaker. Only the selected crisis hot line operator will be able to respond with questions, advice, or "psychological first aid" via the walkie talkie, while the other class members listen and evaluate the operator's performance on their sheets. Five to seven minutes of dialogue is usually sufficient.

Follow-Up Activity

After the hot line dialogue, the performances of both students are discussed by class members through their evaluations and any additional comments by the teacher. Two different students are selected and the activity is repeated. At the end of the period, the assignment for the next class is given: (1) to list all the persons, groups or agencies mentioned, dealing with suicide or attempted suicide (2) to list any verbal or behavioral clues that indicated or implied any self-destructive behavior on the part of the crisis hot line caller.

Health Help Phone Numbers

RICHARD C. HOHN is an associate professor in the College of Health and Physical Education, University of South Carolina, Columbia, South Carolina 29208.

"I'm pregnant!" What a way to start a conversation. The young lady sitting across from me was young, pretty and just about the age of my own daughter. I knew her from my health class but was totally unprepared for such a statement from her. I looked more closely. Her eyes were red and a little wild looking, something like a cornered animal. She wasn't kidding! She had come to me for help. Why me? I'm just a health teacher.

Is it possible that this story could be your story? Are you a teacher, parent, counselor or just a friend to individuals with problems?

The story above is fictional but the situation is not. With that in mind I set out to identity sources which could provide information for health related problems. The sources had to be immediately available, free, and accessible to anyone, anywhere.

After listening to many persons in the helping professions bemoan the lack of immediately available, free information, a search was undertaken to identify as many toll free health related telephone numbers as possible. Outlying health professionals should especially benefit from this information. It is fine to be in a major metropolitan area or near a large university, but it is another matter altogether to be in the middle of nowhere and need immediate up-to-date information. When there is a problem, information is needed immediately, not days or weeks later.

The information in this article can be utilized by students, faculty, parents, and others free of charge. It would seem only reasonable that these numbers be posted in conspicuous places in the school and given to faculty and parents for their use. If you have a question or concern—call!

Finding these helping numbers can be difficult since there is no listing by topical headings in the 800 directory service. The exact name of the service organization must be known.

A possible source of these numbers is the *Toll-Free Digest*. Many university, college, state, and county libraries have this publication in their periodical collection. It can be ordered at a cost of

$1.95 plus 35¢ for postage, from Warner Brothers, P.O. Box 690, New York, NY 10019. The heading "Public Services" has the most number of helping phone numbers.

Ralph Nader's Public Citizens Organization has compiled a list of toll free hotlines. It is also updated and available to the public. Send a self-addressed stamped envelope for each copy to: Hot Line, Public Citizen, P.O. Box 19404, Washington, DC 20036.

Being aware of these numbers and recording new ones in the spaces marked "other" will be helpful. Periodicals and newspapers will have new numbers as they become available.

Health Toll Free Numbers

Sexuality	Major Topic	Hours of Operation

1. Ladies Center Inc.
Florida 1-800-432-0460
Other Continental U.S. 1-800-327-9880
	Abortion
	Birth Control
	Female
	  Gynecological
	  dysfunctions
		9:00 am–5:00 pm
		Mon–Sat

2. National Community Hot Line Pennsylvania 1-800-462-4996 Other Continental U.S. 1-800-523-1885	V.D. Counsel- ing— "Venus"	9:00 am–10:00 pm Mon–Sun
3. Abortion Information 1-800-321-1682 (Will refer to local clinic)		8:00 am–8:00 pm Mon–Sun
4. Other		

Consumer		
1. Action Continental U.S. 1-800-424-8580 Except Washington D.C.	Senior Compan- ionship Peace Corps Foster Grandpar- ent R.S.V.P.	9:00 am–5:00 pm Mon–Fri
2. Consumer Product Safety Commission Maryland 1-800-492-2937 Other Continental U.S. 1-800-638-8326		8:30 am–5:00 pm Mon–Fri
3. Educational Grants Hotline Continental U.S. 1-800-638-6700 For application processing Continental U.S. 1-800-553-6350		8:30 am–5:30 pm Mon–Fri
4. National Solar Heating and Cooling Infor- mation Pennsylvania 1-800-462-4983 Other Continental U.S. 1-800-523-2929		
5. Other		

Runaway		

1. National Runaway Switchboard
Illinois 1-800-972-6004
Other Continental U.S. 1-800-621-4000
	Runaway to give
	  message to par-
	  ents
		24 hr–7 day

2. Operation Peace of Mind
Texas 1-800-392-3352
Other Continental U.S. 1-800-231-6946
	Runaway to find
	  shelter & coun-
	  cil
		24 hr–7 day

3. Parent Anonymous California 1-800-351-0386 Other Continental U.S. 1-800-421-0353	Child abuse	24 hr–7 day
4. Other		

Miscellaneous		
1. Legal aid information 1-800-424-9321		9:00 am–5:00 pm
2. Moving 1-800-424-9321	Interstate Com- merce Commis- sion Hot Line	8:30 am–12:00 pm 1:00 pm– 4:00 pm Mon–Fri
3. Multiple Sclerosis Society Continental U.S. 1-800-243-6000 Except Conn. (for example)		
4. Peace Corps/Vista (See Action) Washington D.C. 254-7346 Other Continental U.S. 1-800-424-8580 ext. 38 and 26		9:00 am–5:00 pm Mon–Fri
5. The Upper Room Living Prayer Center 1-800-251-2468		7:00 am–11:00 pm Mon–Sun
6. Other		

Students Can Have a Say

JOAN L. BERGY, formerly a consumer specialist with the U.S. Food and Drug Administration in Seattle, Washington, became on September 4, 1973 the director of the Seattle Area Office of the U.S. Consumer Product Safety Commission. BARNEY HANTUNEN is the regional public information officer, Public Health Service, Department of Health, Education, and Welfare, Region X, Seattle.

A student voice in government rule-making? A consumer voice in government rule-making? Impossible, you say?

Not really, if you look into a little known publication—the _Federal Register_. Students—consumers—can have an impact on, for example, the selection of the route for the proposed Pacific Crest National Trail, the labeling of cosmetics, and a whole host of planned federal actions which affect all aspects of our daily lives, if they learn about this publication and are willing to take action.

The _Federal Register_ is a legal document published Monday through Friday by the Office of the Federal Register, National Archives and Records Service, GSA, Washington, D.C. 20402.

The _Federal Register_ provides a uniform system for making available to the general public regulations and legal notices issued by the Executive Branch of the federal government. Also included are Presidential proclamations and Executive Orders as well as various federal documents required to be published by Act of Congress.

The format used to present regulations in the _Federal Register_ includes:

...A preamble which reviews the background of the proposal

...A statement of the proposal

...Information on the procedure for submitting comments

...Where comments should be forwarded

...The deadline date for receipt of comments

Following the expiration date the federal agency considers all comments and takes action. The action may be in the form of a "final order" printed in the _Federal Register_, including the effective date for the regulation.

A new requirement now makes it mandatory that every "final order" is to include a summary of the types of comments received and whether the "final order" includes, rejects, or modifies comments received. In any case the "final order" must include the information on which the decision was based.

The process of rule-making begins after Congress passes a law and the President signs it into law. Then, it is the responsibility of the federal agency charged with carrying out the law to prepare appropriate regulations to implement the law. Preparation of regulations is a complex and time-consuming task. However, once that job is done, the regulations are printed in the _Federal Register_.

This is the critical point. Usually 60 days are allowed for comment. This is the time when the student—the consumer—will have the opportunity for reacting to and commenting on the proposed set of regulations. It is also possible to change current regulations by the rule-making process. An individual or any group may petition a federal agency to propose a change in regulations.

The system falls short, however, when consumers do not participate. More often than not the number of comments received in response to _Federal Register_ proposals is very limited.

In March 1973, as an example, FDA published in the _Federal Register_ a proposed change in regulations that would require cosmetic ingredients to be listed in descending order of predominance on labels attached to each cosmetic product. The proposal specified details about the label design, language to be used, size of print, as well as fragrances, coloring, and flavoring used in the product. As of May 1973, the sources of comments were as follows:

...Cosmetic industry and associations—19

...Professional organizations—1

...Universities—3

...Other federal agencies—1

... Organizations—5

... Individual consumers—267

A second example is the proposal to require a warning statement on the labeling of aerosol containers, which was published in the *Federal Register* during March 1973. One of the several proposed warning statements was: "Warning: Do not inhale directly; deliberate inhalation of contents can cause death." As of May 1973, the following summarizes comments received:

... Aerosol industry and associations—21

... Organizations—2

... Universities—5

... Consumers—1

It should be pointed out that the *Federal Register* is not the easiest document for the student or the consumer to locate. It is available from the Superintendent of Documents, Government Printing Office, Washington, D.C. 20202 at a cost of $25.00 per year, or single copies at twenty cents. Most libraries stock the publication. It is also generally available through libraries maintained by federal agencies in the Regional Office cities of Boston, New York, Philadelphia, Atlanta, Chicago, Dallas, Kansas City, Denver, San Francisco, and Seattle.

From time to time proposals published in the *Federal Register* are included as news items in local daily newspapers. However, more often than not very little information is included to guide the student or consumer in submitting timely comments to the appropriate place.

So how can students become involved? How can they gain access to the "system" of federal rule-making? How can they gain a perception of the process which will stand them in good stead as they move from academic community into the community at large?

A prerequisite, of course, is availability of the *Federal Register* in the classroom or the school library. A committee of students might review the *Federal Register* for a period of time in order to select a proposal for class consideration.

Once the proposal is selected, the committee might develop information and perhaps a demonstration project to illustrate to the class what the present regulations are and what changes are contemplated in the proposal. In addition, the students might analyze proposed changes in the regulations and their effect upon industry, the consumers, and others concerned with the subject under consideration.

Upon reaching a consensus and having reconciled various points of view, the comments could be submitted to the agency, as indicated in the *Federal Register,* which has responsibility for preparing the "final order."

The students would then need to develop a follow-up plan to assure continuity in their efforts to observe the final outcome of the process. When the "final order" does appear in the *Federal Register* the students will be in the unique position of comparing their own experience and accumulated materials to the final outcome.

Most important of all, they would have seen, and shared in, the rule-making process. They would, hopefully, have developed a heightened concept of their rights and responsibilities in the American rule-making process.

A Unit for Independent Study in Death Education

JOAN D. McMAHON *is a health education teacher at Thomas Johnson Junior High School in Lanham, Maryland.*

The subject of death and dying is most often rejected by the conscious mind of the American people. Our society is one aimed at the preservation and enhancement of life; denying death and reducing its harshness have helped to cushion the American people's fear of their eventual end.

In coming to grips with the dying process and death, a person may have a better understanding of his own feelings and those of others who are actually experiencing dying and death. Death, for most people who are touched by it, presents a crisis state out of which coping with a new lifestyle becomes extraordinarily difficult. Too many people die suddenly and leave their families totally unprepared to rearrange their living patterns. Learning how to cope with a crisis, then, would appear to aid an individual in his adjustment to such a change as death brings.

A unit for independent study in death education has been prepared; this is an educational method that allows progress at an individual learning rate. It is the primary objective of the unit to help people come to grips with their own feelings and attitudes toward death and the dying process so that life will be more rewarding and enjoyable and death will become less feared.

The unit was compiled for advanced high school or college students or those professionals interested in improving their knowledge of the dying process and death. It was originally developed from suggested course outlines by Daniel Leviton of the University of Maryland, who is cur-

rently teaching a course on death education to over 300 students a semester. In an article in the *Journal of the American College Health Association,* Leviton outlined his topics and speakers for the course.[1] Some of the same general topics are included in this unit. It consists of behavioral objectives, questions to be answered, activities to be performed, and assessment tasks.

UNIT IN DEATH EDUCATION

Prerequisites: Any combination of the following: practicum in counseling; work in crisis intervention centers or on hot lines; course utilizing techniques; course in the psychology of adjustment.

Course Content:

Subunit A: The Taboo of Death
Subunit B: Definitions of Death: Biological, Social, and Psychological
Subunit C: The Crises of Man
Subunit D: Views on Death and Dying
Subunit E: Understanding the Dying Patient or Relative
Subunit F: The Funeral, Burial, and Bereavement: Psychological Implications
Subunit G: Understanding Suicide and Self-destructive Behaviors

Directions: Perform in the following order:

1. Read the behavioral objective
2. Read the required readings
3. Answer the questions listed
4. Perform the activities
5. Perform the assessment tasks

---

[1] Leviton, Daniel, "A Course on Death Education and Suicide Prevention: Implications for Health Education," *Journal of the American College Health Association,* April 1971, pp. 217-20.

Before beginning the course: Answer the following questionnaire and save your responses.

QUESTIONNAIRE [2]

1. When you were a child, how was death talked about in your family?
   a. Openly.
   b. With some sense of discomfort.
   c. Only when necessary and then with an attempt to exclude the children.
   d. As though it were a taboo subject.
   e. Never recall any discussion.

2. To what extent do you believe that psychological factors can influence (or even cause) death?
   a. I firmly believe that they can.
   b. I tend to believe that they can.
   c. I am undecided or don't know.
   d. I doubt that they can.

3. What is your belief about the causes of *most* deaths?
   a. Most deaths result directly from the conscious efforts by the persons who die.
   b. Most deaths have strong components of conscious or unconscious participation by the persons who die.
   c. Most deaths just happen; they are caused by events over which individuals have no control.
   d. Other.

4. Who died in your first personal involvement with **death**?
   a. Grandparents or great-grandparents.
   b. Parents.
   c. Brother or sister.
   d. Other family member.
   e. Friend or acquaintance.
   f. Stranger.
   g. Public figure.
   h. Animal.

5. To the best of your memory, at what age were you first aware of death?
   a. Under three.
   b. Three to five.
   c. Five to ten.
   d. Ten or older.

6. How religious do you consider yourself to be?
   a. Very religious.
   b. Somewhat religious.
   c. Slightly religious.
   d. Not at all religious.
   e. Antireligious.

7. Which of the following best describes your childhood conceptions of death?
   a. Heaven-and-hell concept.
   b. After-life.
   c. Death as sleep.
   d. Cessation of all physical and mental activity.
   e. Mysterious and unknowable.
   f. Other than the above.
   g. No conception.
   h. Can't remember.

8. To what extent do you believe in a life after death?
   a. Strongly believe in it.
   b. Tend to believe in it.
   c. Uncertain.
   d. Tend to doubt it.
   e. Convinced it does not exist.

9. Regardless of your belief about life after death, what is your wish about it?
   a. I strongly wish there were a life after death.
   b. I am indifferent.
   c. I definitely prefer that there not be a life after death.

10. If it were entirely up to you, how would you like to have your body disposed of after you have died?
    a. Burial.
    b. Cremation.
    c. Donation to medical school.
    d. I am indifferent.

11. How much of a role has religion played in the development of your attitude toward death?
    a. A very significant role.
    b. A rather significant role.
    c. Somewhat influential, but not a major role.
    d. A relatively minor role.
    e. No role at all.

12. Which of the following most influenced your present attitudes toward death?
    a. Death of someone close.
    b. Specific readings.
    c. Religious upbringing.
    d. Introspection and meditation.
    e. Ritual (e.g., funerals).
    f. TV, radio, or motion pictures.
    g. Longevity of my family.
    h. My health or physical condition.
    i. Other.

13. Which of the following has influenced your present attitudes toward your own death the most?
    a. Pollution of the environment.
    b. Domestic violence.
    c. Television.
    d. Wars.
    e. The possibility of nuclear war.
    f. Poverty.
    g. Existential philosophy.
    h. Changes in health conditions and mortality statistics.
    i. Other.

14. To what extent has the possibility of massive human destruction by nuclear war influenced your present attitudes toward death or life?
    a. Enormously.
    b. To a fairly large extent.
    c. Moderately.
    d. Somewhat.
    e. Very little.
    f. Not at all.

15. Have your attitudes toward death ever been affected by narcotic or hallucinogenic drugs?
    a. Yes.
    b. I have taken drugs but my attitudes toward death have never been affected by them.
    c. I have never taken drugs.

[2] These questions are taken from the "Death Questionnaire" by Edwin S. Schneidman in *Psychology Today* magazine, © Communications/Research/Machines, Inc.

16. What does death mean to you?
    a. The end; the final process of life.
    b. The beginning of a life after death; a transition; a new beginning.
    c. A joining of the spirit with a universal cosmic consciousness.
    d. A kind of endless sleep; rest and peace.
    e. Termination of this life but with survival of the spirit.
    f. Don't know.
    g. Other.

17. What aspect of your own death is the most distasteful to you?
    a. I could no longer have any experiences.
    b. I am afraid of what might happen to my body after death.
    c. I am uncertain as to what might happen to me if there is a life after death.
    d. I could no longer provide for my dependents.
    e. It would cause grief to my relatives and friends.
    f. All my plans and projects would come to an end.
    g. The process of dying might be painful.
    h. Other.

18. How often do you think about your own death?
    a. Very frequently (at least once a day).
    b. Frequently.
    c. Occasionally.
    d. Rarely (no more than once a year).
    e. Very rarely or never.

19. When you think of your own death (or when circumstances make you realize your own mortality), how do you feel?
    a. Fearful.
    b. Discouraged.
    c. Depressed.
    d. Purposeless.
    e. Resolved, in relation to life.
    f. Pleasure, in being alive.
    g. Other.

20. In your opinion, at what age are people most afraid of death?
    a. Up to 12 years.
    b. Thirteen to 19 years.
    c. Twenty to 29 years.
    d. Thirty to 39 years.
    e. Forty to 49 years.
    f. Fifty to 59 years.
    g. Sixty to 69 years.
    h. Seventy years and over.

21. If you could choose, when would you die?
    a. In youth.
    b. In the middle prime of life.
    c. Just after the prime of life.
    d. In old age.

22. When do you believe that, in fact, you will die?
    a. In youth.
    b. In the middle prime of life.
    c. Just after the prime of life.
    d. In old age.

23. If you had a choice, what kind of death would you prefer?
    a. Tragic, violent death.
    b. Sudden, but not violent death.
    c. Quiet, dignified death.
    d. Death in the line of duty.

e. Death after a great achievement.
f. Suicide.
g. Homicidal victim.
h. There is no "appropriate" kind of death.
i. Other.

24. For whom or what might you be willing to sacrifice your life?
    a. For a loved one.
    b. For an idea or a moral principle.
    c. In combat or a grave emergency where a life could be saved.
    d. Not for any reason.

25. What is your primary reason for the answer to question 24?
    a. To spare my spouse loneliness.
    b. To avoid loneliness for myself.
    c. To spare my spouse grief.
    d. To avoid grief for myself.
    e. Because the surviving spouse could cope better with grief or loneliness.
    f. To live as long as possible.
    g. None of the above.
    h. Other.

26. Has there been a time in your life when you wanted to die?
    a. Yes, mainly because of great physical pain.
    b. Yes, mainly because of great emotional upset.
    c. Yes, mainly to escape an intolerable social or interpersonal situation.
    d. Yes, mainly because of great embarrassment.
    e. Yes, for a reason other than above.
    f. No.

27. Suppose that you were to commit suicide, what reason would most motivate you to do it?
    a. To get even or hurt someone.
    b. Fear of insanity.
    c. Physical illness or pain.
    d. Failure or disgrace.
    e. Loneliness or abandonment.
    f. Death or loss of a loved one.
    g. Family strife.
    h. Atomic war.
    i. Other.

28. Suppose you were to commit suicide, what method would you be most likely to use?
    a. Barbiturates.
    b. Gunshot.
    c. Hanging.
    d. Drowning.
    e. Jumping.
    f. Cutting or stabbing.
    g. Carbon monoxide.
    h. Other.

Subunit A: The Taboo of Death

Behavioral Objective: The student will be able to freely discuss and come to terms with his own feeling concerning death.

Answer the following questions:

1. Why do language barriers exist on the subject of death and dying?
2. How do you perceive death?
3. What euphemisms can you think of to describe death and dying?
4. Do all persons have a negative attitude toward dying?

Activities:

Interview a person about his feeling toward death.

Assessment Tasks:

1. Either talk with someone about your ideas on death or tape record your ideas and replay them.
2. Save the responses that you made to the Schneidman questionnaire.

Subunit B: Definitions of Death: Biological, Social, and Psychological

Behavioral Objective: The student will be able to differentiate between the biological, social, and psychological definitions of death.

Answer the following questions:

1. What is the biological definition of death?
2. What constitutes social death?
3. What constitutes psychological death?
4. How do these definitions interrelate?

Activities:

Upon reading all required readings for this subunit, make a chart depicting the interaction and separation of each definition of death.

Assessment Tasks:

1. Define biological, social, and psychological death as described by the various authors listed in the required readings.
2. Cite three case histories (can be hypothetical) that depict each type of death.

Subunit C: The Crises of Man

Behavioral Objective: Upon identification of the different stages of adjustment to a crisis, the student will apply these stages to death and dying.

Answer the following questions:

1. What are Fink's stages to the adjustment of a crisis?
2. What are Bowlby's stages to the adjustment of a crisis?
3. What are Kubler-Ross's stages of adjustment to a crisis?
4. Do the terminally ill adjust to death and dying according to the stages above?

Activities:

1. Write a story about a terminally ill person who must cope with his own immediate death in terms of Bowlby's model (2 pages).
2. Examine a crisis in your life and determine which model or combination of models approximates your crisis state.

Assessment Tasks:

1. Correlate five patients in Kubler-Ross's book to Bowlby's model as to the stages of adjustment they went through during a crisis.
2. Read one of the following and write a two page explanation of how a character goes through any of the stages mentioned by Fink:
   Death Be Not Proud, John Gunther
   A biography of Eleanor Roosevelt, any author

Subunit D: Views of Death and Dying

Behavioral Objective: Upon examining the required readings on the views of death and dying, the student will be able to briefly explain how death and dying are perceived from the viewpoint of children, adolescents and young adults, the middle aged, the elderly, and the terminally ill.

Answer the following questions:

1. What are the developmental stages in childhood that lead to a mature concept of death?
2. Name three adjustment mechanisms that affect the elderly's attitudes toward death.
3. Name four factors which influence the terminally ill's adaptation or adjustment to their impending death.
4. Do college students perceive death as threatening? Support or refute.
5. How do you feel the middle aged population feels about dying in their prime?

Activities:

1. Create a hypothetical situation concerning a child's reaction to the loss of a pet.
2. Predict how you would react if a person in your family was diagnosed as terminally ill. How do you think they would want you to react?
3. Identify your feelings if you were suddenly faced with the realization that you had a terminal illness.

Assessment Task:

Plan a chart illustrating the various age groups, variables affecting their death attitudes, the behavior that should or should not manifest itself on experiencing a situation involving death, and the views held by each age group on the subject of death and dying.

Subunit E: Understanding the Dying Patient or Relative

Behavioral Objective: Upon learning of the impending death of an individual, the student will be supportive and perceptive of their feelings and needs. The student will also be able to develop strategies for helping the dying patient or relative to cope with death, dying, and bereavement.

Answer the following questions:

1. What emotional and psychological needs should a relative have fulfilled in order to cope with the impending death of a relative?
2. What emotional and psychological needs should the patient have fulfilled in order to cope with his own impending death?
3. Explain the reactions and emotions of those who confront dying daily, e.g., police officers, the mili-

tary, morticians, clergymen, physicians, nurses, etc.

4. How would you feel in the presence of a dying person?
5. Should a patient be permitted to return home to die? Why or why not?
6. Whose responsibility is it to tell a person he is going to die?

Activities:

1. Interview any two of the following concerning their reactions and emotions in observing death and the dying process: police officer, mortician, war veteran, physician, nurse.
2. Identify those factors which cause relatives to desert a dying patient. Do these apply to yourself?

Assessment Task:

Eric is a 14 year old Negro with sickle cell anemia. His family has kept from him all mention of the disease, its symptoms, and its fatal outcome. He has been sleeping a great deal lately and his general condition has been weakening. His teacher has been discussing biology and disease causing organisms with him. He has been asking questions as to whether he has a disease. Eric has noticed that he has little energy and thinks he may have a serious disease but his family has not told him anything. You can perceive that he may ask you what disease he has and what it will do to him.
What needs and feeling do you suppose Eric has? Develop a strategy to cope with Eric's dying with him and his family on your visits.

Subunit F: The Funeral, Burial, and Bereavement: Psychological Implications

Behavioral Objective: This student will be able to evaluate the American grief process and formulate constructive plans for his or a relative's death.

Answer the following questions:

1. Who should make the arrangements for the funeral? Who should be responsible for the final decisions on place of burial, method of body disposal (cremation, burial, etc.)?
2. What constitutes a normal bereavement reaction? What constitutes an abnormal one?
3. What are the religious implications for burial? What are the psychological implications for burial?
4. What grief reactions can be expected upon learning of the death of a child, a teenager or college student, a middle aged individual, or an elderly person?
5. What happens to the family or persons who continue to live after a close friend or relative has died?

Activities: Choose two

1. Consult a funeral director and/or visit his "lab."
2. Decide what your role would be in the death or dying process of mother or father; brother or sister; husband or wife; young child; close friend; acquaintance; and pet.
3. Write your will and go over the legal implications with a lawyer.

4. Plan a financial statement that would include mortgage, insurance policies, children's education, and funeral expenses.

Assessment Task:

Prepare a detailed and operable plan to be used in the event of your death. Include who should be notified of the death, expenses, settlement of the estate, disposal of personal possessions, etc. What is the rationale for your plans and did you account for the needs of the family who would be left?

Subunit G: Understanding Suicide and Self-destructive Behaviors

Behavioral Objective: The student will be able to devise a reference list of persons, groups, or agencies that deal with suicide. He will also be able to identify clues in the individual's behavior that suggest a need for consultation with a professional specialist or a need for other forms of immediate help.

Answer the following questions:

1. Why do children commit suicide?
2. Why do college students commit suicide?
3. What are clues that a person may want to kill himself in the near future?
4. What is crisis intervention and how can it be used in suicide prevention programs?
5. What can you do as a professional or nonprofessional to help an individual cope with his problem?
6. When should you recognize the necessity for professional psychological therapy for the individual? What persons or agencies are available for such referrals?
7. Does a person have the right to take his own life?

Activities:

1. Visit a suicide prevention center or a crisis intervention center that deals with suicide intervention.
2. Contact the Center for Studies of Suicide Prevention, National Institute of Mental Health, Rockville, Maryland 20852.
3. Interview two specialists on campus or in the community who would be in contact with suicide problems: health educator; clergy; sociologist; psychologist; counselor; or health service personnel.

Assessment Tasks:

1. Make a list for your immediate reference of persons, groups, or agencies that you could contact if you face a suicide case.
2. Identify those clues to suicide behavior that constitute immediate help, psychiatric help, or other professional services.
3. Retake the Schneidman questionnaire and compare your responses from your first attempt.

REQUIRED READINGS

Sub-Unit

E
F
1. Bakke, John, "Managing the Fatal Illness," *Northwest Medicine* (1960), 59: 901-904.
An excellent article which clearly discusses the patients' reaction, the physicians' dilemma, the grief reactions, and the family's reaction.

E 2. Beatty, Donald, "Shall We Talk About Death?" *Pastoral Psychology* (1955), 6(51): 11-14.
Do patients want to have their thoughts confirmed about their impending death? The reactions of patients, medical personnel, the family, and the clergy are discussed in relation to the seriously ill patient.

B 3. Beecher, Henry, "Definitions of 'Life' and 'Death' for Medical Science and Practice," in I. Ladimer (ed.), *New Dimensions in Legal and Ethical Concepts for Human Research, Annals of the New York Academy of Sciences,* January 21, 1970, 471-74.
The medical definition of death, long antiquated, is discussed. Reasons for establishing a new criterion for biological death are discussed in light of current medical technology.

G 4. Bennett, A. E., "Recognizing the Potential Suicide," *Geriatrics* (1967), 22(5): 175-81.
Suicide is not produced by external factors—only internal impulses. Elderly persons present special problems. Any indication of depression must be recognized and the conditions treated. Physicians and hospitals must seek to prevent suicide by recognizing and treating potential candidates. Police should be instructed in the handling of suicide attempts, and communities must be educated about suicide and must seek to prevent its occurrence.

D 5. Binger, C., et al., "Childhood Leukemia: Emotional Impact on Patient and Family," *New England Journal of Medicine* (1969), 230(3): 414-18.
Interviews who had lost a child from leukemia were interviewed by a team of four pediatric hematologists, a child psychiatrist, and a social worker. The findings of the team, how these findings have been used in ongoing work with such families, and descriptions of their application by other professionals who face this problem are summarized.

C 6. Bowlby, J., "Processes of Mourning," *International Journal of Psychoanalysis* (1961), 42: 317-40.
The basic psychological processes of mourning are divided into three parts: urge to recover the lost object, disorganization, and reorganization.

A 7. Choron, J., *Modern Man and Mortality,* Macmillan, New York, 1964.
How to cope with the acute awareness of mortality: an "old-fashioned" approach to the question of what death means and "does" to the individual.

D 8. Eisendrath, R. M., "The Role of Grief and Fear in the Death of Kidney Transplant Patients," *American Journal of Psychiatry* (1969), 126(3): 381-87.
Eight out of eleven patients who died following renal transplants were noted to have suffered a sense of abandonment by their families or to have experienced panic. The author discusses these effects through case histories.

G 9. Farberow, N. L., "Training in Suicide Prevention for Professional and Community Agents," *American Journal of Psychiatry* (1969), 25(12): 1702-05.
The author describes the various types of training offered at a suicide prevention center and notes that a primary objective for both public and professionals is to diminish the taboo aspects of suicide.

A 10. Feifel, H., "The Taboo of Death," *American Behavioral Sciences* (1963), 6: 66-67.

A discussion of the contemporary situation in which death is a taboo topic for conversation and investigation.

C 11. ——— "Perception of Death," *Annals of the New York Academy of Sciences,* December 19, 1969, 669-77.
D
The perceptions of death among terminally ill and healthy persons were viewed in the context of religious belief, denial of leaving life behind, professional and social discipline and commitment, and the fear of the unknown. An excellent article.

C 12. Fink, S., "Crisis and Motivation: A Theoretical Model," *Archives of Physical Medicine and Rehabilitation* (1967), 48: 592-97.
Four stages in the process of adjustment to a crisis are discussed with implications to the terminally ill: shock, defensive retreat, acknowledgment of the situation, and adaptation.

C 13. Hackett, T. and Weisman, A., "Denial as a Factor in Patients with Heart Disease and Cancer," *Annals of the New York Academy of Sciences,* December 19, 1969, 802-17.
Denial by the patient as well as disclosure of the illness by the medical personnel make this an article well worth reading for its psychological implications.

F 14. Harmer, R., *The High Cost of Dying,* Crowell-Collier, New York, 1963.
A book directed at the popular market which attacks business methods utilized by funeral directors.

E 15. Herter, Frederic, "The Right to Die in Dignity," *Archives of the Foundation of Thanatology* (October, 1969), 1(1): 93-97.
A positive view of the right of the dying to be informed of their impending death.

F 16. Hinton, John, "Reactions to Bereavement," *Dying,* Penguin Books, Inc., 1967, pp. 167-83.
The rational and irrational emotions associated with death and bereavement are discussed by a psychiatrist who has long been connected with patients suffering from incurable illnesses.

F 17. Jackson, Edgar, "Attitudes Toward Death in Our Culture," in A. Kutscher (ed.), *Death and Bereavement,* Charles C. Thomas, Springfield, 1969, pp. 212-18.
A clear and simple explanation of what the American people do to cope with their grief.

D 18. Kalish, R., "The Effects of Death Upon the Family,"
F in L. Pearson (ed.), *Death and Dying,* Press of the Case-Western Reserve University, 1969, pp. 79-107.
The impact of dying upon the family; first the death of the elderly person, then of the middle-aged person, and finally of the child are discussed in relation to emotions, actions, thoughts, and feelings.

B 19. Kastenbaum, R., "Psychological Death," in L. Pearson (ed.), *Death and Dying,* Press of the Case-Western Reserve University, 1969.
Thanatomimesis, phenomenology, and social death are discussed as relating to psychological death.

D 20. ——— "The Child's Understanding of Death: How Does it Develop?" in E. Grollman, *Explaining Death to Children,* Beacon Press, Boston, 1967, pp. 89-109.
This article examines the stages of development in children toward a mature concept of death.

E 21. ———"Viewpoint: Helping the Patient Prepare for Death," *Geriatrics* (1967), 22(2): 80, 84, 88.
Those who can discuss the prospect of death are

generally more helpful to the patients, who often feel a need to discuss their views on the subject.

A C 22. Kubler-Ross, Elisabeth, *On Death and Dying,* Macmillan, New York, 1969.

The adjustment to a crisis is viewed in stages of denial and isolation, anger, bargaining, depression, acceptance among the terminally ill. The author believes that the dying have a lot to teach the living through various forms of communication. An excellent overview of the psychological implications of death and dying.

A F 23. Lamm, Maurice and Eskeis, N., "Viewing the Remains: A New American Custom," *Journal of Religion and Health* (1966), 5(2): 137-43.

Attempts to demonstrate that viewing of the corpse is objectionable both theologically and psychologically.

A G 24. Leviton, Daniel, "Death, Bereavement, and Suicide Education," in Donald Read (ed.), *New Directions in Health Education,* Macmillan, New York, 1971.

Deals with death education and its goal of helping students understand the relationship of death to life, and life to death.

B 25. Mant, A., "The Medical Definition of Death," in A. Toynbee, et al., *Man's Concern With Death,* McGraw-Hill, New York, 1969, pp. 13-24.

Various medical criteria for determining death are discussed and medical definitions are given in simplistic terms.

D[3] 26. Middleton, W. C., "Some Reactions Toward Death Among College Students," *Journal of Abnormal and Social Psychology* (1936), 31: 165-73.

F 27. Mitford, J., *The American Way of Death,* Simon and Schuster, New York, 1963.

Written for the popular market, this widely discussed book is aimed at exposing alleged malpractices of funeral directors.

G 28. Murphy, G., et al., "Who Calls the Suicide Prevention Center: A Study of 55 Persons Calling on Their Own Behalf," *American Journal of Psychiatry* (1969), 126(3): 314-24.

Fifty-five persons who had called a suicide prevention center on their own are discussed as being psychiatrically ill, attempting suicide before, or in a depressing mood, and therefore needing professional help.

D 29. Nagy, M., "The Child's Theories Concerning Death," *Journal of Genetic Psychology* (1948), 73: 3-27.

Written compositions, drawings, and interviews were employed in an effort to find out what children from 3-10 years old think about death.

A 30. Peniston, D. H., "The Importance of Death Education in Family Life," *Family Life Coordinator* (1962), 11(1): 15-18.

The subject of death as taboo is discussed. Its relevance as subject matter is projected as a positive learning experience which should be looked at with an open mind by both children and adults.

G 31. Ross, Mathew, "Suicide Among College Students," *American Journal of Psychiatry* (1969), 126(2): 220-25.

A survey of college student suicides which indicated that there is an unusually high rate of suicide among college students. The author believes that college student suicide is predictable and preventable and

---

[3] To be read with possible implications for today's college population.

that early recognition and prompt appropriate treatment are excellent preventive efforts.

A G 32. Schneidman, Edwin S., "You and Death," *Psychology Today* (1971), 5(1): 43-45, 74-80.

This is a report on a questionnaire given to college students. The student responses to the questionnaire are extremely interesting.

E 33. Schoenberg, Bernard, "The Nurse's Education for Death," in A. Kutscher (ed.), *Death and Bereavement,* Charles C. Thomas, Springfield, 1969, pp. 55-74.

This chapter within a book is devoted to factors which determine how the nurse copes with the patient. Her reactions to death are discussed in an interesting manner.

E 34. Senescu, Robert, "The Problem of Establishing Communication With the Seriously Ill Patient," *Annals of the New York Academy of Science,* December 19, 1969, 696-706.

The needs of the patient are often ignored because the medical personnel don't pay enough attention to the emotions of the seriously ill.

B 35. Smart, Ninian, "Philosophical Concepts of Death," in A. Toynbee, et al., *Man's Concern With Death,* McGraw-Hill, New York, 1969, pp. 25-35.

Dying and death are discussed as distinguishable phenomena, and the emotions experienced when facing death are examined philosophically.

B 36. Still, Joseph, "We Need To Know Not Only When Human Life Ends But Even More Important, When It Begins," *Archives of the Foundation of Thanatology* (Summer, 1970), 2(2): 66-74.

Life and death are described as occurring in levels: cellular, organ, organismal, psychic, and vegetative. Interesting interpretations on the definitions of life and death can be questioned by the reader.

E 37. Strauss, Anselm, "Family and Staff During Last Weeks and Days of Terminal Illness," *Annals of the New York Academy of Sciences,* December 19, 1969, 687-95.

The focus is on the emotions and actions of the family and nursing staff in the dying process of an individual.

B D 38. Swenson, W. M., "Attitudes Toward Death on an Aged Population," *Journal of Gerontology* (1961), 16: 49-52.

Attitudes toward death can be measured objectively. Such a measure has indicated that religious subjects are less likely to fear death than nonreligious subjects.

E 39. Zinker, Joseph and Fink, S., "The Possibility for Psychological Growth in a Dying Person," *Journal of General Psychology* (1966), 74: 185-99.

To help evaluate the meaning of death in human existence, it was deemed important to study the behavior of individuals most intimately concerned with death, specifically, those who are dying. Maslow's formulations of need hierarchy are used as the framework for conceptualizing growth versus decline. Both psychopathology and the capacity to transcend, to love, and to create are present in the dying person.

G 40. "One Every Twenty Minutes," *Medical World News* (1967), 8(14): 73-78.

An epidemiological study of suicide and the factors that cause people to turn to suicide as an escape technique.

TEACHING IDEAS

Death and Dying

Put a Little Life in Your Death

CHARLES R. O'BRIEN *is a graduate student in the Department of Health and Physical Education at Bowling Green State University, Bowling Green, Ohio 43403.*

During the past years in health instruction, there has been a major drive by educators to include the topic of death and dying in the curriculum of their institutions. One of the many reasons for this impulse is because of the changes in society. With these changes, death has been taken out of the family structure and been replaced by "outsiders."

Years ago death was a significant aspect in the foundation of the family. An individual was born, lived, and died at the same location. Death at this time was an experience which was cherished by the family, friends, and individual religious beliefs. At the present time however, people tend to hide their children from the reality of death and pay others to take the burden off their hands. Recently this factor has presented numerous mental problems for a number of Americans. Some of these problems have resulted in child runaways, suicide, breakdown of religious beliefs, and have forced changes in individual life patterns. Because of these and other reasons, the public and the education profession think it is necessary for the topic of death to be included within the educational structure.

Since death education is beginning to be included in many school systems, it has created problems such as: what content areas should be included in a death unit and how are the content areas to be taught? Some major personal questions should be examined before you attempt to construct your unit on death. The first question should be: do you know *your* philosophy on death?

Research indicates that there are two basic philosophies dealing with death. In both of these philosophies the primary concern is awareness. The reason for this is that by being *aware* of death the individual may be able to see the full life cycle and make the proper choice of philosophies to complement the individual's behavioral needs.

Philosophy 1 is death fear. In this philosophy people have such a fear of death that they change certain patterns in their life to accommodate this fear. By doing this they minimize the risk of death and also many of life's pleasures.

Philosophy 2 is death acceptance. In this philosophy individuals understand and accept the reality of death. Through acceptance of death within themselves, they lead their lives in whatever way they wish, and accept the final outcome of these actions.

The second personal question one should ask is: Do you fear death? If the answer to this question is yes, take another look at this fear, determine if you fear death or if you fear dying. These are two terms which sometimes are used synonymously, but are they really? Death means *the end of life* whereas dying is *the process of death*. There are many ways of dying such as through disease, aging, and accidents. With an individual there is only one death. This death may come in two speeds: slow as in disease, old age, and pollution; fast as in accidents, suicide, war, and domestic violence.

Once you have gone through this self-realization process, you should be able to see one of the basic reasons for teaching about death—the students' wellbeing. Death education could be an important aspect of every individual's life. Death as we know it now is something which happens to everyone, but is something we have little control over. Individually we may be able to put off death through exercise, diets, and good health practices, but death itself remains the same.

Now that you are aware of your views on death you can start examining topics which will be included in the death unit. The following topics can be included.

1. Religious beliefs
2. Rituals
3. Stages of dying
4. Types of funerals
5. Insurance
6. Attitudes toward death and dying
7. Heaven-hell concept
8. Death philosophies
9. Euthanasia (direct-indirect)
10. Types of dying (physical-mental-social)

Once you have your topics planned, find the teaching activities to complement your lesson. Here are just a few.

1. Visit a cemetery
2. Visit a funeral home
3. Invite guest speakers (coroners, doctors, lawyers)
4. Make poems
5. Make up tombstones and epitaphs
6. Write an obituary
7. Write out wills
8. Make up a life inventory
9. Role play
10. Interview students
11. Look up laws on death (state and taxes)
12. Crossword puzzles

To help with the classroom activities, teaching techniques like small group discussions, debates, and problem-solving seem to be enhanced by the use of recordings. Below is a list of records which pertain to death education and help stimulate student participation.

1. "Ohio"-Neil Young
2. "Life in the Bloodstream"-The Guess Who
3. "Unborn Child"-Seals and Crofts
4. "Imagine"-John Lennon
5. "Talisman"-The Guess Who
6. "Fiddle in the Sky"-Seals and Crofts
7. "Changes IV"-Cat Stevens
8. "Follow Me"-Seals and Crofts
9. "Better off Dead"-Elton John
10. "Heaven Only Moved Once Yesterday"-The Guess Who

In today's society we find it morbid to discuss and think of our own death. By not discussing death, we place it in the closet hoping it will not become a reality we will have to face. A unit on death would make possible a needed discussion to help eliminate the problems discussed earlier. It would also help students understand the full meaning of life and bring out the necessity of understanding death.

DEATH EDUCATION:
An Integral Part of School Health Education

Darrel Lang is health coordinator for the Turkey Valley Community Schools, Jackson Junction, Iowa, and a member of Iowa's task force for comprehensive school health education.

School health education is a continuous process which enables the student to assume individual responsibility for developing and maintaining personal behaviors which promote total wellness.[1] If this goal is to ever be achieved, death education needs to be integrated into the school's health curriculum.

Six years ago a death occurred in my family and this was my first close contact with death. I felt totally inadequate and concluded that many of my students probably fit into this same model. To counter this inadequacy, I integrated a death education unit into our mental health strand for the secondary level.

Before I could develop a proper unit that would adequately serve the majority of my students, it was necessary to conduct a ten-question attitude/information inventory. From this inventory, I was better able to understand my students' feelings about death.

The inventory is self-explanatory and gave me a fairly good perspective on the approach I should take with my students towards death education. The following is a copy of the unit in death education that I feel has adequately served my students.

Attitude/Information Inventory

1. To what extent do you believe in a life after death?[2]

   Male   Female
   A. Strongly believe in it.
   B. Tend to believe in it.
   C. Uncertain.
   D. Tend to doubt it.
   E. Convinced it does not exist.

2. To what extent do you belive in reincarnation?

   Male   Female
   A. Strongly believe in it.
   B. Tend to believe in it.
   C. Uncertain.
   D. Tend to doubt it.
   E. Convinced it cannot occur.

3. How often do you think about your own death?

   Male   Female
   A. Very frequently (at least once a day).
   B. Frequently.
   C. Occasionally.
   D. Rarely (no more than once a year).
   E. Very rarely or never.

4. What does death mean to you?

   Male   Female
   A. The end; the final process of life.
   B. The beginning of a life after death; a transition, a new beginning.
   C. A joining of the spirit with a universal cosmic consciousness.
   D. A kind of endless sleep; rest and peace.
   E. Termination of this life but with survival of the spirit.
   F. Don't know.

5. What aspect of your own death is the most distasteful to you?

   Male   Female
   A. I could no longer have any experiences.
   B. I am afraid of what might happen to my body after death.
   C. I am uncertain as to what might happen to me if there is a life after death.
   D. It would cause grief to my relatives and friends.
   E. All my plans and projects would come to an end.
   F. The process of dying might be painful.

Death Education Unit—Outline

Day 1 —Introduction to death education.
Survey on death.
Drawing: Visual Impression of Death.

Day 2 —Vocabulary of death.
Funeral customs around the world.

Day 3 —Protestant-Catholic View of death.
(Minister & priest guest lecturers).
Other religious views of death.

Day 4 —Class collage on life and death.

6. When you think of your own death (or when circumstances make you realize your own mortality), how do you feel?

                Male   Female

A. Fearful.
B. Discouraged.
C. Depressed.
D. Purposeless.
E. Resolved in relation to life.
F. Pleasure in being alive.

7. If you had a choice, what kind of death would you prefer?

                Male   Female

A. Tragic, violent death.
B. Sudden but not violent death.
C. Quiet, dignified death.
D. Death in a line of duty.
E. Death after a great achievement.
F. Suicide.
G. Homicidal victim.
H. There is no "appropriate" kind of death.

8. What are your thoughts about leaving a will?

                Male   Female

A. I have already made one.
B. I have not made a will, but intend to do so some day.
C. I am uncertain or undecided.
D. I probably will not make one.
E. I definitely won't leave a will.

9. To what extent do you belive in life insurance to benefit your survivors?

                Male   Female

A. Strongly believe in it; have insurance.
B. Tend to believe in it; have or plan to get insurance.
C. Undecided.
D. Tend not to believe in it.
E. Definitely do not believe in it.

10. What are your thoughts about funerals?

                Male   Female

A. Feel they are very important for the bereaved.
B. Tend to feel they are valuable.
C. I am uncertain or undecided.
D. Definitely do not believe in them.

Day 5 —Filmstrip, *Living with Dying*,[3] on how America lives with death.

Day 6 —Five stages of death, grief and bereavement.

Day 7 —Film: "*What Man Shall Live and Yet See Death*[4], Part I.

Day 8 —Film: *What Man Shall Live and Yet See Death*[4], Part II. Drawing students' own tombstone and writing epitaphs.

Day 9 —Pictorial report on epitaphs taken from cemeteries. Death-related music.

Day 10—Group reports on death
1) Life insurance
2) Military view on death
3) Medical examiner
4) People who have been brought back to life.

Day 11—Fantasy exercise on death.[5]

Day 12—Field trip to funeral home.

Day 13—Positive-negative euthanasia.

Day 14—Explaining death to children.

Death has been a fascinating subject that people have always questioned. Through a thorough unit on death education, many questions and thoughts about death may be answered. It is hoped this approach would better educate our youth and eventually our society. We all should have a better understanding of death, for we *ALL* will face it some day.

1. *Definition of Comprehensive School Health Education*, Iowa's Task Force on Comprehensive School Health Education.

2. *Perspectives on Death Student Activity Book*, David W. Berg, George G. Daugherty, 1972., p. 2-4, Arlington Press, 201 Eighth Ave. S., Nashville, Tenn. 37207.

3. Sunburst Communications, Pleasantville, N.Y. 10570.

4. Area Educational Agency, Film's, Inc., 1972.

5. *Psychology of Death & Dying*, John C. Morgan, Richard L. Morgan, Westinghouse Learning Press, Sunnyville, CA.

Death and Dying

A Teaching Strategy on Tragedy

CONNIE JO DOBBELAERE *is a graduate
assistant at Bowling Green State University, Department of Health and Physical
Education, Bowling Green, Ohio 43402.*

"Mary's life seemed to be at a perfect
point! She was 16 years old, pretty, in-
telligent, enthusiastic, a varsity cheer-
leader, and had just been elected
homecoming queen for her high school.
She had a happy home life, with two
brothers, four sisters, two parents, and
a dog named Brownie. Mary loved life
and had everything to live for. On a
clear night in March, she was driving
home from work, just getting ready to
make the left hand turn off of Highway
617 into her driveway—when from
nowhere a semi-truck started to pass
her on the left. Mary died on March 23,
1976."

A similar tragedy may happen at any
time in your community or school system. The question is, how do we prepare our students to handle the death of
a friend or loved one properly? Is there
ever a proper way to handle this situation?" Death 40 to 50 years ago was accepted as a natural culmination of life.
However, today Americans try to cover
it up and pretend that when death does
occur they will be able to accept it. This
idea has not proven to be valid in recent
years. There appears to be an inescapa-
ble need to furnish our youth with a
more comprehensive view of what
death really means, how they can cope
with a death when it occurs, and why it
is important for them to carry on and
live a more fulfilled life.

A death education unit taught in a
health class needs to be implemented
for the benefit of each student. If death
is accepted as a natural part of life, an
inevitable event in all existence, then we
will be able to stress the importance of
living life to the utmost for *today!* The
main objective, it seems evident, is for
the death unit to emphasize the need to
develop in each individual a crisp zest
for every undertaking, day-to-day, that
one can. Life is rich in varied opportunities and the mission is to find and perceive each and every advantage that

arises. We teach death in order to better
live and understand the total process of
life!

A Tragedy Strategy

Once the need for a unit on death
education has been established, the next
problem a teacher faces is just exactly
how to introduce the unit into the classroom. One teaching strategy, which
proved to be very functional in past
health instruction and upon which this
article is based, used a questionnaire entitled "You and Death," by Edwin
Shneidman.[1] It contains approximately
72 questions which were condensed to
40 for class purposes. In essence, it en-
tails answering the questions in an attempt to identify and clarify students'
feelings and conceptions on death. The
questionnaire proved to be a thought
provoking and discussion stimulating
technique to introduce the death unit.

For a more complete and interesting
discussion of the questionnaire, the
students were instructed to mark a star
by the most thought provoking questions; an "S" by those which most surprised them; a "T" beside the questions
about which they would really like to
talk with someone; and an "MI" in front
of those questions they would like more
information on as they went through
the test. These marks pinpointed the
areas of most interest for the ensuing
discussion. They also symbolized to the

students where their ideals and values
needed to be researched and clarified
further.

Four of the 40 questions that were
clarified at some length in the classroom
are discussed here. They exemplify the
type of discussion that was carried on as
a result of the questionnaire.

The first question seemed to influence
the way in which the students answered
the rest of the questionnaire: to what extent do you believe in a life after death?
a. strongly believe in it; b. tend to believe in it; c. uncertain; d. tend to
doubt it; e. convinced it does not exist.

Some students were confused about
their feelings on the subject and therefore seemed to have a great deal of
trouble completing the test. However,
others answering the question either
completely affirmatively or completely
negatively had little trouble with the
test. By discussing the question in
greater detail it appeared that most of
the students felt more at peace with
their own feelings towards the subject
and felt more open about their convictions because they found out that they
were not the only ones who had trouble
with the subject.

A second question prompting interest
tried to clarify situations in which one
would give up one's own life: For whom
or what might you be willing to sacrifice
your life? a. a loved one; b. an idea or
moral principle; c. in combat or a grave
emergency where a life could be saved;
d. not for any reason.

Most of the students had a great deal
of difficulty imagining sacrificing their
lives for anyone or anything. Most of
the members enjoyed their present
lives. However, they all agreed that
they would probably change their
minds if they were confronted with a
real life situation involving one of these
choices.

Another thought provoking question
had to do with the actual date of one's
death: if it were possible, would you
want to know the exact date on which
you are going to die?

The catalyst of this discussion was
supplied by one student's statement
that "if I were told that I was going to

live to be at least 40 years old, I would live life to its fullest and try to experience all that life affords and not wait for old age to do the things I've always dreamed of doing." Others responded that they would definitely not like to know when they were to die because it was a fearful subject for them and they would rather not think about it. Still another response was shared with the class by a student stating that it really doesn't matter to him whether or not he knew because his religious faith was so strong and he was so satisfied with his present life that anytime death came he would be ready.

Conclusions made from this question helped students to answer and discuss a fourth question: What effect has this questionnaire had on you? a. it has made me somewhat anxious or upset; b. it has made me think about my death; c. it has reminded me how fragile and precious life is; d. no effect at all; e. other effects (specify).

Most of the students responded to the question by either marking "b" or "e." The questionnaire did make them think about their own death but it also made them deliberate about their feelings on suicide. It also brought suppressed feelings out into the open and helped them to be more content with their ideas on death and dying.

As we discussed the whole topic of death once more in the summary, they felt also that they could have responded "c" as well. The discussion of death did remind them of the pricelessness of a fulfilled life and forced them to reevaluate their personal lives at the present time.

Strategy Evaluation

As a final evaluation of this experience, the students filled out a sheet of open-ended statements. These evaluations proved even more valuable than the discussion. It helped students to be more understanding of each other's personal feelings and views on death and the pricelessness of a fulfilled life.

The students were given no directions on the proper way to complete the statements and thus were forced to answer them with their own unique perceptions of the total experience. In sharing some of their answers it is my hope that each reader will see how successful

the strategy proved to be for each participant. Some of the answers from the students follow.

I learned that . . .
—life, though often taken for granted is temporary, and protection of same, even promotion of same is of number one priority.
—"death education" can be an interesting topic if taught with the objective of living life better for now.
—I am able to stand firmly convicted to the belief in life after death—not fearing death as we know it here on earth.
—I am satisfied with my life and death concept.

I want to . . .
—find out more information about the stages of life when one's attitudes toward death change.
—live what life is afforded me to its fullest, but regretfully must adjust to constraints (some of which may be unnecessarily self-imposed).
—live my life to the fullest and when death comes, I hope to accept it gracefully and it accept me the same way.
—live daily with the attitude that today is my only opportunity to tell others why I don't fear death.

I hope that I . . .
—can live life productively, yet joyously—and never stray from the sense of perspective that enables me to "always smell the flowers . . ."
—can develop sharper opinions on some of the questions I was unsure of.
—if I discover I am scheduled to die soon, I can lead exciting final days and not spend my last days pouting and cursing my destiny.
—live to be a ripe old age!!

I was surprised to see that . . .
—some people didn't want to give their lives for others.
—when confronted with the possibility that even I might consider suicide, I really could not think of the way in which I would take my life.
—I don't have very many strong convictions about my attitude toward death.
—some refuse to seek the full life.

I was glad to see that . . .
—my religious faith is strong enough to answer most of these questions with ease.
—I was consistent in my thoughts on death.
—I did have to think as a result of this questionnaire about my feelings on death.

—others believe in God and put their trust in His promise for eternal life.
—Many treasure *living*—not as solely based on survival ethics, but on a *fulfilling* basis . . . "I want all from life that is good and beautiful."

I want to remember that . . .
—today may be my last—I need to keep a smile on my face and a rainbow in my heart!
—no matter what else I learn through my educational career I am sure to remember *today!*
—whatever I do with my life—the only important thing is to die with Jesus controlling my heart.
—death is not the end!
—life has order, peace, love and total appreciation of nature."

Death education can be a mind-expanding unit if taught with the objective of getting the students to learn to accept and understand death and to think of it as an inevitable end to life, as we know it here on earth. When they can accept this phenomenon, they can develop a more meaningful opinion about the necessity to *live* life to the utmost and to instill in themselves a zeal for a more fulfilled life.

It is vitally important that one learns that one does not have to wait for tragedy before confronting the fundamental and ineluctable questions related to death and dying with which one may be confronted. The requirement here is for one to be willing to participate and learn to understand and accept death as a natural part of all life.

---

[1]Edwin Shneidman, Center for Advanced Study in the Behavioral Sciences, in consultation with Edwin Parker and G. R. Funkhouser of Stanford University, "You and Death," *Psychology Today*, Communications Research Machines, Inc.; Del Mar, CA, August 1970, pp. 67–72.

Suggested Readings

Hendin, David. *Death as a Fact of Life.* Warner Paperback Library: New York, 1973.

Hendin, David. *Concerning Death: A Practical Guide for the Living.* Earl A. Grollman, ed. Beacon Press: Boston, 1974.

Kubler-Ross, Elisabeth. *On Death and Dying.* MacMillan: New York, 1969.

Kubler-Ross, Elisabeth. *Death the Final Stage of Growth.* Prentice-Hall, 1975.

Stanford, Gene and Perry, Deborah. *Death Out of the Closet.* Bantam Books: New York, 1976.

Health or Hazard? A Post-China Syndrome Game

Moon S. Chen, Jr.

Moon S. Chen, Jr. is an assistant professor of health education at Ohio State University, 215 Pomerene Hall, 1760 Niel Avenue, Columbus, Ohio 43210.

How important is it to teach about ionizing radiation or noise protection or industrial safety? For most students, these three topics seem remote and removed from the classroom. However, the movie, *The China Syndrome*, made the Three Mile Island incident and the hazards of radiation hauntingly realistic. Students and teachers in the Harrisonburg area were undoubtedly affected and students elsewhere certainly felt curiosity and a need to know more facts. What better place to bring together the topics of radiation and health hazards of the working environment than in an environmental health course or in a unit on environmental health? And how better to make learning more fun than with a game?

Fun and success with such a game, called "Health or Hazard?", are attributed to proper orientation and to student involvement and discovery. Orientation to the game consists of a cognitive introduction to the basic forms of radiation (e.g., ionizing—alpha, beta, gamma rays, and non-ionizing—microwaves) and how to use time, distance, and shielding for protection. A cognitive introduction to health hazards of the working environment should cover the detrimental effects on humans of noise, dust, gases, and toxic liquids. Protection measures would include environmental manipulation, medical surveillance, management decisions, and personal protection. Students should be taught to adapt such principles to specific hazards (that is where much of the learning occurs).

Following cognitive input, the teacher should divide the class into three equal-sized and intellectually-matched groups. One group will be student referees with responsibility for awarding points and making decisions regarding disagreements between sides. Their preparation will consist of correctly matching hazards with proper health protection methods.

The two other groups will be competing teams. Each team should prepare itself independently. Based on the cognitive information given in class, each team should prepare an array of "offensive" hazards and an arsenal of "defensive" health protection measures. Each hazard and each health protection measure should be written on a separate index card large enough so that it can be read across a classroom.

The spirit of competition between the two sides fosters a spirit of cooperation on each side. Team members naturally help each other in learning the associations between hazards and the proper health protection.

Competition begins after about fifteen minutes of preparation. Each side alternately chooses a player from the opposite team to "challenge." Each challenge is considered a "round." Each team alternately assumes an offensive and defensive position.

During the round the offensive player chooses a hazard with which to "attack" the defensive player. The hazard is hidden from view until the offensive and defensive players face each other in the front of the classroom. The defensive player brings his arsenal of methods. On a signal from the judge, the offensive player flashes his hazard. The defensive

player has fifteen seconds to respond by showing the card with the correct health protection measure against that hazard. If the correct health protection measure is not on one of the defensive player's cards, the defensive player has the same fifteen second time limit to write the proper health protection on a separate index card. No coaching from teammates is allowed.

A score results when either side wins a "round." Decisions regarding which side wins will be made by the student judge for that particular round. The student judge must decide whether the defensive player's response is correct and made within the fifteen-second limit. (The time should be kept by another judge.) If the defensive player displays the correct response within the time limit, the defensive side scores a point. If not, the offensive side wins a point. The first team to win a predetermined number of points wins.

For greater variety and excitement, more than one hazard can be introduced at one time, forcing the defensive players to respond more quickly. This game can be played at the pace of the students. It is fun, exciting, and a harmless way to learn health protection measures against radiation and hazards of the working environment.

Nuclear Power Debate

Bruce G. Morton is an assistant professor of health education, at Temple University, Philadelphia, PA 19122.

The nation is entering its second decade of crisis over energy resources and energy consumption. Gasoline has more than doubled in price in the past two years. The rising price of home heating oil threatens the health and welfare of poor people who are unable to pay their bills. Congress is considering a proposal to relax environmental standards for strip mining and air pollution emissions from coal-burning power plants. Rampant inflation, partly caused by skyrocketing energy costs, threatens public health as government slashes social programs to balance the budget.

Concurrently, the long term commitment of the nation to the nuclear pathway to energy independence is being reconsidered. The major accident at Three Mile Island, together with the less publicized but nonetheless serious incidents at Browns Ferry, Chalk River, Rocky Flats, and Idaho Falls, have thrown a pallor over the once rosy future of nuclear power. At this writing only one state in the country (Tennessee) is now willing to accept radioactive wastes for storage and disposal. Among the general public, concerns about radiation, the potential for sabotage and the contribution of nuclear power technology to nuclear arms development, have grown dramatically in recent years. Among those who define themselves as environmentalists, opposition to nuclear fission power is virtually unanimous.

But there are two sides to each of these questions. Proponents point to the impressive safety record of nuclear plants. They argue that without nuclear power, electricity would be much more expensive than it is now and the air would be more polluted from coal-fired power plants. They contend that there are benefits and risks to every energy alternative and nuclear benefits far outweigh the risks.

In a course I teach on health and the environment I attempted to broach the problem of presenting the conflicting information which clouds the nuclear question, by organizing a debate in which the students assumed the roles of various interested persons as described below. The purpose of the exercise was to provide the students with the opportunity to try on various viewpoints regarding nuclear power in a simulated real life situation. First I provided the students with readings from a range of perspectives; then I presented the pros and cons of each of the relevant issues in as unbiased a manner as possible. A general discussion ensued. Emphasis throughout was placed on determining the credibility of the information and on the subsequent identification by students of the issues, facts and feelings salient to their attitudes and values toward nuclear power. I found a plethora of biased materials written for the lay public from the local electric company and from one of the local anti-nuclear groups active in my community. I augmented this with academically credible sources. (A list of references is available on written request).

The procedures for the debate that I have found to be most valuable are as follows:

1. During the class session prior to the scheduled debate, present or discuss the issues with reference to the articles which the students should already have read. Next, break the students into groups as per the directions below.

2. At the beginning of the second class, just before the debate, give each group 10-15 minutes to compare notes and ideas, and select one person to serve on the panel.

3. Solicit a volunteer or assign someone to be moderator. Charge this person with the responsibility for limiting the time for each presentation and facilitating the democratic opportunity for everyone who wants to speak at least once.

4. Ask those not on the panel to assume the roles of concerned citizens who have the right, and who will be given the opportunity, to ask questions or make statements.

5. Plan 30-40 minutes for the debate including questions and comments from concerned citizens not on the panel.

6. After the debate, open up the class to general discussion and give people the opportunity through discussion and voting to identify the issues, concerns and feelings most important to them, and to clarify and affirm their personal values with respect to nuclear power.

Directions to Role Players

You are a participant in a discussion among local residents and interested persons concerning the proposal by the electric company's directors to build a nuclear power plant in your neighborhood. Each of you may select one of the following roles but there must be at least one person for every role. For the purpose of the exercise attempt to assume the arguments of the role assigned as you perceive they would be. Each person on the panel will have a maximum of five minutes for an initial statement after which there will be time for rebuttal and open discussion.

Participants

Sal/Sally Slick is the electric company's spokesperson. She/he is an outstanding proponent of nuclear power whose special talent is putting the levels of risk posed by nuclear power into perspective with other risks from automobiles, coal mining, natural disasters, cigarette smoking, etc.

Bert/Bertha Booster is the Chamber of Commerce public relations person. Although this character may be either for or against nuclear power, she/he is indefatigable in boostering local business.

Conrad/Connie Concerned is a local resident who is the parent of two children who go to school in the vicinity of the proposed power plant.

Alan/Alice Academic is the local university scientist who is concerned with the balanced presentation of the facts. She/he will often bring out the other side of the argument so that everybody will be apprised of all the facts. She/he likes to put things in the perspective of risks and benefits.

Ed/Edna Ecology is a local environmental activist who is deeply concerned about the ecology of the river on which the plant is proposed to be built as well as a number of other environmental problems.

Be conscientious about limiting the time for each panel member to present and rebut. The purpose of the exercise is to get a range of viewpoints out in the open, not to resolve the issues or to judge the presenters. The 10-15 minutes in groups before the debate assures that each panelist will have a few good points to make, and is itself a good exercise in information sharing. However, you may want to provide the moderator with a few leading questions just to get the discussion going should it come to a standstill. Usually, the reverse occurs— it is hard to limit the debate. The role playing seems to provide many students with a comfortable vehicle for interaction, and the instructor with a method for examining a controversial health concern.

Environmental Health

Health and Safety Education from the Trash Can

I. CLAY WILLIAMS is an associate professor of health education at Bowling Green State University, Bowling Green, Ohio 43402. JUDITH K. SCHEER is assistant professor of health education at the University of Toledo, Toledo, Ohio 43606.

As educators, we constantly dream of ways to obtain effective visual aids to help us develop concepts; however, the difficulty of getting school monies appropriated for visual aids to enhance classroom presentations too often confronts us. I am going to share a secret of how to cope with, even *enjoy,* two problems of our everyday existence—teaching on a shoestring budget and taking out the trash! The trash can offers unlimited potential for collecting an abundance of effective teaching aids. My recent practice of accumulating discarded items provides a wealth of invaluable materials for the classroom that we can use effectively to develop important health and safety concepts.

In my collection is a necktie which is ripped and tattered. It makes me think back to early spring, several years ago. I was itching to get my boat in the water so, on returning home from church, I announced that anyone who wanted to go to the lake should be ready to leave in five minutes. My wife objected saying that I had promised to build some kitchen shelves for her and that I was not leaving the house until the job was done. Needless to say, I was in no mood to build kitchen shelves! Rushing like a madman, I started to cut a board with the circular saw and the next thing I knew, my tie was tangled in the saw blade which was rapidly approaching my throat! Looking at the mutilated tie and thinking about the close call, I suddenly realized what a perfect visual aid this would make in teaching about hazard potential of various items of clothing. I saved the tie and it became the first of many items in my "trash can collection."

A plastic cup brings to mind a personal example of how an accidental poisoning might occur. I wanted to make a smoking machine out of a liquid detergent bottle so I went into our kitchen, grabbed the soap bottle, and poured its contents into a plastic cup, placed the plastic cup on the window sill and began making the smoking machine.

About a week later, Tom was making lemonade for the twins and found only one clean glass in the cupboard. Looking around, he spied the plastic cup on the window sill and filled it with lemonade for Robby. Robby took a big drink and started to cough and choke tearfully. His mother came running in and said, "What's the matter? Is your lemonade too sour?" She took the glass from him and sampled it herself to see what was wrong, and she's been blowing bubbles ever since! This is an excellent example of how poisonings occur in the home! We are fortunate that the glass didn't contain drain cleaner, automatic dishwasher detergent, or other

toxic substances which would have caused extensive tissue damage. By this example, we can learn quite a lesson about proper storage.

Other trash that can be used to teach about poisons is abundant. A paint can with a "lead-free" label is an appropriate visual aid when teaching about lead poisoning. A rusty, swollen or dented food can might be the focus of questions designed to stimulate an awareness of food poisoning.

Once your trash collection becomes well known, others will bring you items and stories to add.

"I'd like to donate this to your trash collection," said one of my students as he handed me an old extension cord. The cord was peeling and cracked and dried out with wires exposed. He had used this under the carpet for several years. Instead of just telling students not to run extension cords under rugs, this cord can show how friction will break down the insulation. When students were asked to suggest ways that the cord might have become so abused, they told of pets which had chewed through extension cords and about times when heavy duty appliances were used on light duty extension cords causing the cord to deteriorate. One of the values of utilizing items from the trash can is that they act as discussion stimulators providing students with opportunities to share personal experiences.

One such experience involved a handmade sweater which our twins decided to use as a replacement for their lampshade when redecorating their room. The light bulb encrusted with charred wool and the tiny sweater with a hole the size of a grapefruit tell the rest of the story. Luckily, it was a wool sweater! Had it been made with synthetic yarn, it could have caused a fire instead of smoldering as it did. With the sweater and light bulb or other wearing apparel the concept of flammability in clothing could be explored.

The topic of home fires is rich with bizarre stories. This past summer, I heard a lot of commotion in the kitchen, so I came running in from the back yard and saw flames shooting out from behind the refrigerator. The coils on the back of the refrigerator had come into contact with the plug; over a period of time, vibrations had caused the coils to cut through the insulation. The melted plug is a good reminder that we should regularly check our electrical appliances.

In my trash collection I have a dish towel that touched the lower heating element in the oven. A section of it burned away when it was being used as a pot holder and the unsuspecting cook had a fire.

As a child, you probably enjoyed playing with tape measures. Jeff was no exception. While watching TV, he was reeling out a tape measure and watching it spring back. As he reeled it out, the end dropped between a chair and the far wall; Jeff flew out of his chair, eyes like saucers and hair standing on end. The metal tape had come into contact with the prong of a lamp plug which was not all the way into the receptacle. The other end hit the aluminum frame around the sliding glass patio door. At the contact points, the tape melted and charred. Jeff's tape clearly illustrates how seemingly harmless activities can be dangerous if the right conditions exist.

The average person can do little to prevent the unexpected; however, a safety conscious individual can take measures to guard against common hazards. When purchasing electrical

appliances how careful are you to look for the Underwriters Laboratory (U.L.) label? When I found a battery charger at an unbelievably low price I looked on the display card and found the U.L. label. It wasn't until sometime later that I realized the U.L. approval applied only to the cord and plug—not the battery charger. How often we have been led into a false sense of security by not reading the fine print!

Items like the extension cord, sweater, refrigerator plug, tape measure, and U.L. labels are discarded daily. Alert your friends and students to save these types of items for you. It has been our experience that students are much more willing to listen, share, and remember examples of home hazards than they are to memorize lecture notes of do's and don'ts.

Hundreds of suffocations occur in homes each year. Students become directly involved when I introduce the subject of suffocation by placing a plastic bag over my head. I demonstrate when plastic bags are and are not dangerous. A plastic bag, tied in knots, will illustrate the proper method for its disposal.

My mother-in-law receives shirts from the cleaners in plastic bags which

she uses for jobs around the house. When the twins were three, they discovered those bags in Grandmother's kitchen. They were just the right size to get over their heads. I happened to walk in just as Robyn pulled one down over her eyes and nose. Had she been more successful, she would have been in

great danger of suffocation. A larger plastic bag in my collection was on a crib mattress at a hotel which could have tragic consequences if tired parents don't take time to check for such hazards.

Many other household helpers can be hazards. We all know that power tools should be handled with great respect, but often there is a tendency to abuse or be careless with "everyday" tools. You probably have a screwdriver with a blade that chipped because the tool was used as a chisel, a crowbar, or something else for which it wasn't designed. When there is finally an opportunity to tighten a screw, there's not enough blade. As you apply pressure, trying to turn the screw there is danger of per-

sonal injury as pressure causes the broken blade to slip from the screw head.

Another example is my 98¢ bargain hammer which was designed for light use such as driving tacks or small nails. When the kids decided to build a fort in the back yard, they used my hammer to drive spikes. Half the spikes went in crooked so they tried to pull them out. All of a sudden the claw broke, and there was a flying missile that might have put out an eye. These would-be-architects also damaged my hammer so that the head would no longer fit. To avoid upsetting me, they left it on the workbench just as they had found it, saying wrong. A week later, as I was working on a project the hammer head flew off and sailed

through the garage window onto the hood of my car. Are you saving your plastic bags, broken screwdrivers and hammers as aids in developing concepts relating to hand tools and home safety?

Annually, hundreds of youngsters are fatally injured as a result of home firearm accidents. Many of these accidents occur because youngsters don't understand the danger of firearms. It is not uncommon for children to consider .22 caliber guns as toys because of the small size of the cartridge. In an attempt to make students appreciate the destructive capabilities of a small bore gun, I showed them a soft drink can which was shot with a .22 hollow point.

This mutilated metal creates a lasting impression when used to illustrate the damage a .22 caliber bullet could inflict on a human body. Gunshot wounds can also be explored with x-rays obtained from a radiologist. My x-ray of a skull that has been penetrated by BB clearly illustrates the importance of safe gun handling.

These items are examples of numerous objects that can be recycled from the trash to the classroom. As educators know, the more we can do to allow students to identify with our subject matter the more we can enhance the learning process. By using common items of junk as a focal point for discussing real life situations, teachers can help students develop important concepts concerning their own health and safety. Tight school budgets and rising inflation might be just the motivating factors to encourage rummaging through the trash for classroom stimulators.

Ecology Games

Environmental Health

RONALD W. HYATT is assistant professor, Department of Physical Education, University of North Carolina, Chapel Hill, North Carolina 27519.

Ecology is currently a "hot" topic in health education courses in colleges and high schools. The topic is relevant, the subject matter is current, abundant resource material is available, the mass media are active on the topic, public and private agencies are concerned, and the students are involved in chang-

ing attitudes and legal approaches toward ecological matters. Still, the competent health education teacher, with all of this support, seeks fresh ideas in teaching ecology. Your department editor has experimented with a learning approach in ecology which is current, innovative, educationally sound, economical, appropriate to several school levels and allows for student creativity. This method is the game simulation technique, which allows students to create their own ecology games with ecology problems and solutions presented in the games.

The rationale for using this instructional technique is, to some extent, based on the games theory which was developed in the 1960s at Johns Hopkins University and other institutions. The games simulation theory, which has been used extensively in social studies, political science, and consumer education, uses reproduced materials,

documents, historical events, and historical persons in a game setting with the rules and regulations for the game based on the possibilities found within that game. Rules and regulations are based on the many combinations which have or could occur in the interplay of people, places, and events. Learning opportunities for the student are many, varied, and allied in theme. Creative situations are different for each student and each group. In brief, the game simulation method produces an excellent learning situation. Granted, this approach is rather a simple one, but it can be modified for use on the college and high school levels and, perhaps, the junior high school level merely by making local classroom adaptations.

It is noted that several commercial games are marketed in the area of ecology. *SMOG, Litterbug,* and *Cleanup* are good examples of these. *Pollution,* a commerical product using game simulation, is suitable for use with junior high school students through adults. The learning experiences described here are different from the commercial games in several respects. Some of these differences are as follows:

1. The students provide the input and knowledge necessary to develop their own game.

2. The game conditions are current.

3. The game situation can be scaled to local problems.

4. The creative aspect is present.

5. Small group work is educational and fun.

6. Decisions must be made by the players which are relevant to their needs of the moment.

Materials Needed

Few materials are needed, and they are inexpensive. Six or eight pieces of cardboard, scissors, felt tip pens or crayons, glue, and scrap paper are sufficient. (Recycling is practicing what you teach!)

Class Organization

Group leaders are appointed, and six to eight students are grouped in the areas of population, water, air, noise, and others as class size warrants. An extensive bibliography is handed out several classes prior to this experience. Students are oriented as to the purpose

of the class: to develop a game related to their area of interest. This game must contain rules and regulations, include choices and chances, and involve a decision-making process. Some of the rules may be preplanned, or they may be developed on the spot. The model of monopoly may be used where dice are rolled or number cards may be developed as a means for the students to travel around the board, encounter the different situations, and experience learning opportunities. Chance cards are placed at appropriate areas, and students have to decide on a course of action. (For example: A student draws a

card and has the choice of additional waste controls in the company in which he owns stock, or he has an increased dividend of two dollars. What will he/she take?) Who wins the game and how winners are declared are parts of the game which the group must establish in their rules and regulations.

Starter Ideas

In case your students need kick off ideas, here is an approach one class used.

NOISE POLLUTION: A player starts out with normal hearing. He moves and lands on a square of rock music (3 decibels hearing loss), construction (−5 decibels), or sonic boom (+ nervousness to your physical condition). Chance cards might be safety legislation, adding carpets and drapes in house, etc.

The teacher can use starter ideas to get the groups rolling, but normally a good introduction to the problem is sufficient.

Desired Outcomes

The following teaching points are among those that should be made forcefully and vividly while ecology games are being used.

1. The "random chance approach" to ecology matters, as expressed by the dice or cards, is insufficient in real life. Cooperative planning must take place if we are to win the ecology game of life.

2. There is a total involvement needed of legal methods, legislative processes, citizenship practices and concepts, industrial concerns, religious beliefs and practices, and genuine concern about people and our environment.

3. An understanding of the interrelationships of ecology systems and subsystems is a prerequisite to effective action.

4. Careful selection in the means of correcting the different ecology problems, so as not to produce additional problems of ecology, is important.

5. There should be a greater concern and knowledge about ecology with its problems and promises.

The kind of game simulation and game development outlined briefly here has worked for this teacher on the college level. The students like it, and its use creates an effective learning situation. Other health teachers on different levels in other locales might well use this approach to help their students learn more about ecology.

Guidelines for a Recycling Project

George H. Brooks is assistant to the dean of the University of Northern Colorado Graduate School and chairman of the Greeley Committee on Environment.

Health educators and their students may become involved in local environmental action by helping to establish a community newspaper recycling program. One such program has been successfully operated since July 1971 by the Greeley (Colorado) Committee on Environment. The committee, appointed by the city council in 1969, originally consisted of about a dozen members—businessmen, housewives, teachers, and faculty members. Other members have been added, including a staff member of the local newspaper—a recent journalism graduate, keenly interested in the committee's work, whose added publicity efforts have greatly helped the success of the project.

The committee decided to undertake a newspaper recycling project after learning that 50% or more of the volume of municipal solid waste is made up of paper and paper products, and that about half of that volume consists of newspapers and magazines. They contacted a paper salvage company in Denver, which assured the committee that they would purchase the paper they collected.

A subcommittee was appointed to find a building to serve as a central collection center. In a long, unfruitful search they found building owners reluctant to permit storage of newspapers because of the potential fire hazard, or desiring to secure a long-term tenant. They investigated the possibility of securing a railroad car on a convenient siding, but learned that a car couldn't be spared. A local trucking firm, learning of the project, offered to spot a semi-trailer in a local shopping center parking lot on collection day, then haul the trailer to the paper salvage company in Denver. Permission was gotten to use the parking lot area —far enough away from the main parking lot traffic pattern, yet permitting smooth in-and-out traffic flow along both sides of the trailer. Arrangements were made with the local police department for traffic control and with the city street department for portable barricades to channel traffic flow along both sides of the trailer.

The second Saturday of the month was selected and publicized as collection day. The Committee on Environment loaded the trailer that first Saturday, while a subcommittee sought volunteer groups to furnish labor for loading in subsequent months. The first day's collection yielded 27 tons. Seeing what the collection could amount to, the committee decided to share the monetary return from the sale of paper with the groups which offered to help —one-third to the committee, one-third to the morning volunteer group, and one-third to the afternoon group. The news media carried the story of the committee's plans for continuing the paper collection on the second Saturday of each month. Volunteer groups, wanting to earn money for their projects, were soon put on a waiting list as groups were assigned collection days several months in advance.

A telephone answering service agreed to receive calls from aged persons and others unable to bring their papers to the collection center. Trucks and station wagons, furnished by members of the groups working at the collection center, collected papers from callers. Most people who wanted pick-up service made their calls ahead of the 10 a.m. deadline on collection day. There was little cause for concern over abuse of the service.

The Committee on Environment hopes that Greeley will soon combine its trash collection with recycling on a city-wide basis. However, though the technology is available for such an undertaking, the market for recycled materials needs to be expanded. Even paper collection alone is not yet feasible on a city-wide basis; the paper salvage company says it would be unable to handle all of Greeley's paper along with all the other paper delivered to its docks.

Greeley's Committee on Environment can boast of a great deal of first-hand experience with what has become a widely accepted but not always practiced dictum: man must live with his environment, not despoil it. People will cooperate, if properly informed and motivated with sound, well-planned projects.

Here are some suggestions for those who want to start their own recycling project.

A market for the materials to be recycled is a must. The company accepting secondary materials must be notified in advance of the start of your project.

Have adequate transportation available. Greeley's first Saturday collection filled a 40-foot van type semi-trailer. Every Saturday since, two trailers have been needed; in March 1972 a third truck was partially filled.

Advise city officials and the police department of your project.

Publicize each collection day, taking into account the different deadlines of daily and weekly newspapers and radio and television stations. Announce and adhere to opening and closing hours; remind people not to leave materials at any other time. Include phone numbers of key committee members and answering service, if any. Give clear instructions on how materials are to be tied, bundled, or boxed.

Liability insurance is a must.

Have adequate workers on hand —a minimum of 10 or 12— during all collection hours. At times even that may not be enough, though at other times it may be too many. Workers may need gloves for handling paper bundles. Lifting bundles by the heavy cord soon wears blisters on tender hands.

Someone should be responsible for receiving the checks by mail from the company purchasing the papers or other materials. A home address or Post Office box may be used. The same person should be authorized to write checks to the volunteer groups who furnish labor for your project, and should keep records of names and mailing addresses.

Easy Ways of Getting into Trouble When Teaching Sex Education

GLEN G. GILBERT is associate professor of health education, Portland State University, School of Health and Physical Education, P.O. Box 751, Portland, Oregon 97207.

During my career as a health educator I have observed or have had related to me numerous stories of problems teachers have encountered while teaching sex education. Without exception these teachers have been well meaning and have had the best interest of their students at heart. Poor judgment on their part, however, has often resulted in placing their sex education programs in jeopardy; many supporters of sex education have become nonsupporters because of incidents involving poor judgment. It is the hope of this article that such error can be minimized by calling them to the attention of present and future teachers of sex education. The list offered here is by no means complete as teachers are constantly finding new ways to get into trouble. Here are a few easy ways of getting into trouble teaching sex education.

1. *Teaching sex education with inadequate background.* Sex education is one of the few areas where teachers are actually held accountable for what they teach. Teachers of almost any other subject area can have some poor days of teaching and as long as they maintain order it is unlikely they will ever be chastised for their teaching. Let teachers of sex education make an error and you can bet they will hear of it. It isn't that they shouldn't be held accountable, because they certainly should, but that such accountability is rare in education and a major challenge for sex educators. There are few nondedicated teachers teaching sex education for long, as it is a great deal of hard work. It requires a thorough background in the subject matter— university courses, seminars, and/or a great deal of solid reading. Making content errors in this subject will quickly result in lack of credibility with students, parents, colleagues, adminis-

trators, and will certainly draw the fire of the anti-sex education group.

2. *Keeping your principal or administrator in the dark.* It is imperative that your principals and administrators be apprised of what is happening in your classroom. If you really wish to get into trouble with administrators put them through a couple of late night phone calls from irate parents concerning sex education material or projects which they know nothing about. It is highly likely you will also be blessed with a call from that administrator. Keeping the appropriate administrator up to date, for some, will mean just a statement that you are now studying sex education. For others it will mean detailed lesson plans from which you are not to deviate.

3. *Giving "secret" lessons.* Another surefire way to get into trouble is to have secret lessons with your students. Just make a statement such as "Today's lesson is just between you and me—it is our little secret" and you can be certain many parents will hear of it. You have no business teaching material that you cannot defend.

4. *Violating district or school policy.* This is clearly a violation of your responsibility as a teacher. Curriculum guides are set up to give you parameters to work in, and in a general sense reflect the wishes of the community. You should stay within those parameters no matter what "you know is good" for your students. If you don't agree with the curriculum you should certainly work to change it, and a great many curricula need improvement. Until you get it changed, however, you are legitimately bound by contract to reflect the existing curriculum.

5. *Using poorly constructed home made materials.* Parents especially do not find a poorly constructed penis model or free hand drawings of genitalia amusing. Remember that you are dealing with their children. Giving a homework assignment of freehand drawings of the male and female genitalia may seem innocuous, but many a parent has noted that their daughter drew an erect penis and wondered where she got her model

image. Using anatomical drawings is certainly a legitimate exercise, but have them duplicated for your students.

6. *Using questionable language.* Slang terminology is often all students know of reproductive anatomy and physiology. Students should not be reprimanded for using such terminology unless they use it on purpose to create a disturbance, but they should be tactfully taught the correct terminology. Teachers who feel they must use such terms generally to "get on their level" may soon be on their level equally unemployed.

7. *Not previewing films or materials.* There should be a district committee to approve films, and you are courting disaster if you use films not on the approved list. It is always wise to preview films, but in sex education it is essential. I will never forget an acquaintance of mine who was not teaching health education by choice, and consequently used a large number of films. He ordered the district approved-for-high-school film, "The Story of Eric" (an excellent film on Lamaze childbirth), for his class. As the film progressed he was not prepared for the scene of actual childbirth. He jumped in front of the projector, and his class witnessed a childbirth in vivid color on his white shirt! He had not previewed his film and was not trained or willing to discuss childbirth.

8. *Not being prepared for opposition.* Most programs that are properly established suffer little opposition, as the vast majority of Americans support sex education, but numerous programs have been attacked. All teachers should be able to verbalize the need for sex education when called upon and should anticipate such encounters. Do not respond with hostility or contempt. Parents will have honest questions and they deserve sincere well-documented answers.

9. *Teaching by the joke.* Several instructors have gotten into trouble by telling or allowing students to tell "off color" jokes in the classroom. Teachers telling inappropriate jokes can give the sex education classroom an improper

atmosphere for such an important subject. One local high school teacher got into trouble by leaving his classroom for a long distance phone call. In his absence a student leader was left in charge, who allowed jokes to be told. It was an all male class and the jokes soon got off color and deeper in raw sexual expressiveness. One male not accustomed to hearing women discussed in such terms left the room in tears.

10. *Setting unrealistic goals.* Many programs have been set up with goals and objectives to eliminate VD, divorce, etc. Such programs are doomed to failure. A good example of this is when a program sets out to lower the VD rate. When a good sex education program is established, the VD rate often goes up! The reason for this increase is that people recognize signs and symptoms and go in for treatment. At a later date the rate may go down.

11. *Forcing teachers to teach sex education.* Mandating that all teachers should teach sex education is ludicrous. Forcing teachers to teach in any area they don't wish to teach is unwise. Such action frequently leads to poor quality education, and in sex education that can lead to disaster. Many teachers will never be comfortable teaching sex education. Such unwilling or embarassed teachers can easily be turned to an anti-sex education position by such forced compliance.

12. *Letting personal bias overly influence teaching.* Everyone knows what normal sexual behavior is—it is the way *they* behave. This erroneous belief of major consequence is often carried into the classroom and can be devastating. The advocate of open marriage, marriage at all costs, or any other particular lifestyle has no business preaching it in the classroom. We are all biased. Recognize that bias and be careful not to try to convert your students.

13. *Using inappropriate guest speakers.* The selection of guest speakers must be done with great care. Inviting right-to-life groups to class with brutal pictures can be a traumatic experience for students. Certainly the anti-abortion groups should have the right to express their point of view, but you as a teacher have the right and the responsibility to screen how it is done. Inviting homosexuals to a junior high or high school class is another example of an easy way to get into trouble. Certainly they should have the right to express their opinion, but the problem thus created might jeopardize a total program.

14. *Citing personal sexual experience.* It seems hard to believe that teachers need to be reminded that this is not okay, but it still occurs. Do not let students push you into revealing your personal life. It simply has no place in the classroom.

15. *Using nonapproved questionnaires of students' sexual experiences or attitudes.* It may seem to you that finding out what is actually going on with your students is a good place to start your program, but your principal or administrator is likely to think differently. Remember that such questionnaires may be construed as a reflection of the performance of the school or district as a whole. Be certain to clear all such questionnaires beforehand. They may provide useful information, but be careful they don't cost you your job or hurt the reputation of your school.

16. *Leaving nonapproved reading matter out for public view.* It is of course appropriate for you as a teacher to read anything you wish, but remember that the district has approved materials for use with students. Do not leave nonapproved matter out where a student might pick it up or where an outsider might view it. There is an excellent paperback on birth control and STDs (sexually transmitted diseases) entitled *Intercourse Without Getting Screwed* which is a valuable resource. Many parents, however, may not find the title amusing if they happen to walk by and view it on your desk.

Please ask yourself if you are unnecessarily endangering your sex education program. Sex education is far too important to be eliminated or watered down because of mistakes in judgment. Remember, sex education is one of the few areas of education where teachers are truly held accountable for their teaching. Making errors in teaching history, English, or any other subject seldom results in chastisement, but make an error in teaching sex education and you may be looking for a new line of work.

Readers are advised to review the NEA publication *Suggestions for Defense Against Extremist Attack: Sex Education in the Public Schools,* by the Commission on Professional Rights and Responsibilities, Washington, D. C. Readers might also wish to consult with local universities, the American Association of Sex Educators, Counselors and Therapists (AASECT) and the Sex Information and Education Council of the U.S. (SIECUS) for appropriate courses in sex education in their locale.

Three Teaching Strategies

A soap opera, a silent walk, and a puzzle help present the facts about sexuality in a way that is comfortable for both teacher and students

FLORENCE J. SNARSKI and CECELIA A. LYNCH are health educators teaching sex education courses at Scotch Plains-Fanwood High School, Scotch Plains, New Jersey.

Prior to using any teaching method, the instructor must carefully examine the philosophy of his/her course as well as the role of the teacher in the classroom. Our basic philosophy is that sex education is the study of me-you-us. Sexuality cannot be separated as a discrete, identifiable part of us. It permeates every aspect of our behavior. Therefore, as sex education teachers, our role is to help our students learn more about themselves and others. In our classroom, we consider three general areas of self: physical-psychological-societal. We do agree there is more to the total person than these aspects; however, time and situation limit content offerings.

As health educators, we have a part in the growth of our students in an area that is extremely interesting to them and most humans. It could be so easy to slip into the same techniques for all our classes. Therefore, we strive to use different techniques to meet the needs of each student and the different personalities of each class. Effective teaching strategies can be as important in sex education as solid factual information.

In determining teaching strategies, we feel there are basic questions to ask yourself:

What do my students want to learn?

What do I want my students to learn at this time?

How can I involve my students in this learning? How am I most comfortable dealing with this? Do I have limitations in this area?

Once these questions have been considered, the instructor can institute techniques that will deal with the three areas mentioned: physical-psychological-societal.

YOUR OWN SOAP OPERA

Purpose: In sex education there is a need to explore societal expectations versus individual values.

Objectives

To explore varied life styles.

To become aware of society's expectations for behavior.

To explore alternate modes of responses to life situations.

To stimulate creative thinking.

To illustrate the dynamics of day-to-day living experiences as they influence our choice of behavior.

Procedure: Divide class into groups of four, providing for male/female input in each group, if possible.

Each group is instructed to create a couple, giving biographical structure to the couple, such as age, education, jobs, familial relationships, status of couple's relationship, socioeconomic position, how did they enter each other's life, etc.

After the groups are given about 20 minutes the fictitious couples are presented to the class with a discussion of each couple as they relate to variabilities that may influence their relationship, the future of the relationship, the permanency, and what kinds of needs this relationship meets for each partner.

AWARENESS WALK

Purpose: A relevant task of the sex education teacher is to provide for exploration of differing values among the students. An underlying factor in developing these attitudes stems from previous learning experiences. Though we share some commonalities, we behave individually.

Objectives

To illustrate individual, divergent perceptions in reaction to identical environments.

To stimulate an understanding of one's own learning processes.

To provide insight into one's own responses or lack of responses.

To provide communication channels relevant to different attitudes about sexual behavior.

Materials

Paper/pencils

Ditto slips reading: "We are on a classroom experiment. We are not allowed to talk to you. Please check with my teacher (Name) for further information. We are timed so please do not delay us. Thank you."

Procedure: Divide class into groups of four. Instruct students they are to be nonverbal until further notice.

Each group is to take a walk in and around school environs deciding nonverbally where they are to go and planning to return to the classroom in 10 minutes. One member of the group will take a ditto explanation should anyone confront them in the halls. They are instructed to open their senses to everything around them on the walk.

Start the groups a minute or two apart so that one group moves out of sight before another begins.

Upon returning to the classroom, each student (still nonverbal) is asked to write down all the things they became aware of on their walk.

When all groups have finished writing, allow five minutes for each group to share perceptions among the group and then form a large circle to discuss the differences in perceptions and translate the responses to variances in behavior.

Conclusions: You will find yourself referring to this exercise many times in subsequent classes to explain differences in behavior. This exercise provides a subtle learning experience which requires teacher skill for translation into application.

LIFE PUZZLE

Purpose: A crucial building block for open communication in sex education is the establishment of a "working vocabulary." An innovative review of anatomy and physiology of the male and female reproductive systems is through the LIFE puzzle.

Objectives:

To display knowledge of terms and definitions of reproductive systems—male and female.

To provide student participation in general review.

To determine areas requiring further clarification.

Materials:

Large box
LIFE puzzle

To prepare LIFE puzzle:

1. Cut four letters—L I F E—out of large pieces of construction paper (24 x 36). For coding purposes and ease of instruction, a different color is used for each.

2. Divide each large letter into segments, with each segment containing two pieces which have been cut into interlocking irregular pieces. The number of total segments of all letters is determined by usual class size so each student has at least one puzzle part. Also to be considered are total number of terms and definitions for review.

3. On one half of the segment the anatomical term is written and on its interlocking half is placed the definition.

4. Make a master layout designating what terms are on the appropriate large letter for instructor's reference.

5. Place all puzzle parts into one large box.

Procedure: Students select puzzle parts containing a term or definition pertaining to the reproductive systems. Each student must find partner with corresponding term or definition. Partners present term/definition to the class and then place their portion on the floor to put puzzle together, eventually spelling out the large word LIFE.

Note: Depending upon class size and time schedule, this activity may require more than one class period to complete.

Conclusion: At the end of the lesson, the students have defined their terms. But this can also be used to illustrate the balance of life, that all these terms together "spell" life creating as well as sustaining.

TEACHING IDEAS

The Implementation of Contraceptive Education

WARREN L. McNAB is an assistant professor of health education at the University of Houston, 3801 Cullen Blvd., Houston, Texas 77004.

Eleven million teenagers in the United States today are sexually active;[1] 20% use contraceptives on a regular basis.[2] The unfortunate result of this behavior is indicated by one million unwanted pregnancies, higher fetal and maternal death risk, increased number of female school dropouts with a greater risk of unemployment, forced marriages, and a higher suicide rate among expectant teenage mothers. These statements certainly indicate the need for contraceptive education as a primary means of prevention.

Contraceptive education is not only providing information and services to prevent teenage pregnancy. It is also education for young men and women who later in life may want a family and will need to select a method of birth control that will allow them to plan for a wanted pregnancy. In addition, contraceptive education teaches those who do not want children to select a method which will allow them the nonparent life style they wish to live. It is imperative that we, as educators of sexuality, reinforce our cognitive objectives and principles through relevant learning activities which will enhance the total sexuality and decision making skills of today's young people. With these concepts in mind the following learning activities are structured for three different target groups—the junior high school student, the senior high student, and the parent.

Don't Clown, Burst Misconceptions—Grades 7–9

This activity is effective as a *culmination* to a basic introduction of birth control methods, functions, and knowledge dispelling misconceptions. In front of the class is a large, colored drawing of a clown. From his hands, strings project to different colored balloons. Above his head is the caption: Don't Clown, Burst Misconceptions! Inside each inflated balloon is a misconception about contraception; underneath each balloon on construction paper the same size as the balloon is the reason why the statement in the balloon is a misconception.

The activity is started when the teacher asks students of different teams to correctly spell words related to contraception. Examples are diaphragm, endometrium, intrauterine, lactation, gynecology, ovulation, etc. If the student spells the term correctly his team receives two points. If the student misspells the word he must come to the clown drawing, burst a balloon, and explain why the statement in the balloon is false. A correct answer is worth two points. If the student cannot explain why the statement is a misconception, he opens the construction paper balloon and reads the correct answer to the class. An example of a misconception is: A woman cannot become pregnant while lactating. The answer disproving this misconception is: 20% of nursing women who do not use a birth control method become pregnant, and ovulation precedes menstruation. Reaching a certain point total can be the end of the game.

Projected Future— Grades 10–12

Individually students are given the following hypothetical situation: If you and your husband/wife have decided not to have children for a while, or have decided upon a nonparent lifestyle, what contraceptive method would you use to prevent pregnancy? Justify your choice based upon the physical, mental/emotional, and social implications of the contraceptive on your health. For this exercise list the following headings in separate columns: problem; alternatives; consequences; decision.

The problem is selecting a contraceptive. Individually the students fill in the categories based upon knowledge re- ceived in class and their own feelings about the different methods. There are several contraceptive choices or *alternatives,* and there are many different physical, mental/emotional and social *consequences* that will ultimately affect an individual's decision. After individual selection, groups of four or five students can share their contraceptive choices and justify their selection with others in the group. The teacher and class can then identify similarities and differences of contraceptive preference based upon the physical, emotional, and social factors influencing or prohibiting one's contraceptive choice.

Dear World—Parents

This activity is to help facilitate communication between parents and their sons and daughters. Parents individually and/or collectively decide how they would answer the following letter:

> Dear World:
> I'm a parent with two beautiful teenage children. Tom is sixteen and Christine is fifteen, and both are dating regularly. While I certainly respect and trust them, I want to talk to them about the "facts of life," contraception, and responsible behavior. I know I am much too late, but they seemed to grow up so fast! How can I go about talking to them and what should I say?
>
> Signed Tongue Tied Parent

Following the parents' individual responses they can collectively talk of the problem, what their response would be, and how they would go about talking to a son or daughter. From this involvement parents can share ideas and discuss other ways to open family communication channels about human sexuality.

During our lives we are continually making important decisions based upon what we as individuals feel is best for our own sexuality. Learning activities involving the cognitive and affective domains which help students make decisions based on their own perception of a given situation, reinforces individual responsibility which is paramount to contraceptive education and preventive health.

Bibliography

Guttmacher Institute, *11 Million Teenagers,* Planned Parenthood Federation of America, New York, 1976.

Byrne, Donn. "A Pregnant Pause in the Sexual Revolution," *Psychology Today* 11:2 (July, 1977) pp. 67–78.

Pregnancy—A Gaming Technique

EDWARD T. TURNER is professor and the coordinator of graduate studies, Health, Physical Education and Recreation; and teacher of human sexuality, Appalachian State University, Boone, North Carolina 28608.

Gaming techniques are becoming more and more a part of our educational classroom teaching methods. With the greater use of games numerous companies have been manufacturing simulations and games for use in the classroom. These games are very good but they have two drawbacks: they are expensive; and they may not meet the specific needs of a given teacher's class situation. Games and simulations can be easily thought out and constructed by any interested teacher in order to meet his/her own individual classroom needs. Pregnancy is one such game which was designed for use in a senior graduate college class on human sexuality. The game has been quite successful in that it has greatly enhanced learning through competition in a fun sense. The largest problem in constructing any game of this type is getting your thoughts together on just what you wish the game to encompass. The following construction steps are helpful hints for putting together a board game, such as Pregnancy.
1. Select your topic or area.
2. Collect ideas which you feel should be included on the topic.

3. Select appropriate format for the physical layout of the game.
4. Place the needed information in the appropriate places on your board.
5. Construct your boards with colored tag board or poster board and cover them with clear contact paper in order to increase their longevity.
6. Select equipment including markers, dice, spinner, and decide on the number of players.
7. Select rules and interpretations—play the game a number of times, revise your rules as needed.
8. Mimeograph enough copies of the game and rules so that each member of the class has an individual copy.
9. Revise rules and procedures and adjust game as necessary.

Pregnancy Game—The Layout (See sample drawing and cards)
The Doctor Draw and Conception cards are cut out of heavy paper, and stacked on the board face down. On the back of each card is printed Doctor or Conception.

Pregnancy Rules
Players—2 to 5 players per board. Coed group preferred.
Equipment — board, markers and one die.
1. Decide who is to go first.
2. Each player rolls the die and moves his/her marker, beginning on Start Fin.

3. When a player lands on a space he/she must read aloud the message written on that space. Discussion among group members ensues. This is an important part of the learning concept of the game.
4. If a player lands on Conception or Doctor Draw he/she selects the top card, reads it aloud, and makes the move. The group discusses it.
5. Each player follows the same procedure.
6. The first person to reach the newborn happy face is the winner. The exact number must be rolled on the die in order to reach Baby Happy Face. If another number is rolled the player must wait until the next turn to complete the game.

7. Other players continue until all have reached the end with the total group, including those already finished, still responding in the discussion.

This is just one type of board game that a teacher can construct at a minimum cost. Any other health topic or any other area can lend itself to a similar game. The time and effort in formalizing the idea is well worth the positive learning which ensues.

CONCEPTION CARDS

Abdomen begins to enlarge during the third month—buy loose fitting clothes—Take an EXTRA TURN.

Morning sickness—nausea during the morning hours from 6th to 14th weeks. MISS ONE TURN.

More frequent urination. Uterus is pushing against bladder—MISS ONE TURN in order to buy extra toilet tissue.

GO BACK 4 SPACES

DOCTOR DRAW CARDS

Egg not implanted in uterus properly—go back to nearest conception.

Miscarriage—Natural abortion up until 6th month of pregnancy —go to emergency room—miss one turn then go to StartFin.

Cesarean birth—incision in wall of abdomen in order to deliver baby—stay still and miss three turns.

Artificially induced labor— oxytocin—take two extra turns.

EMERGENCY—Go To Emergency Room and miss two turns

CONCEPTION CARD

4th week—Food passing from mother to embryo

2nd week—2 membranes form around embryo—an inner and outer. Fluid between them is amniotic fluid—structure is known as bag of waters.

DOCTOR DRAW

Implantation of zygote in uterus wall—6th to 9th day

Float Trip in uterus for several days

Rapid Cell Division and Zygote Becomes similar to small hollow ball

Three day trip down the tube

Newly fertilized cell is called zygote

Doctor's Office

Doctor Draw

One Sperm of 2-400

End of 1st month Embryo is ¼" long, heart beating 65/B/pm, eye, ears, & nose begin to form, & (Doctor's office)

End of 2nd month Embryo is 1" long. Large head, nervous system functioning, embryo starts to move this point on embryo known as fetus

Rest— Doctor's Office

Emergency Room

CONCEPTION

PREGNANCY

DOCTOR DRAW

Labor Stage 3— immediately after delivery for 10 min. vigorously ends with passing of placenta (afterbirth)

Breathing begins within one minute, feet grasps and baby

DOCTOR DRAW

End of 3rd lunar mth— Fetus is 3" long, teeth forming under gums, fingers and toes, bare thin nails and sex is distinguishable.

End of 4th lunar mth— Fetus is 6¼" long, body covered with downy hair, skeleton is hardened, and mother may feel fetus movement.

CONCEPTION CARD

End of 5th lunar mth— Fetus is 9½" long, more movement, heartbeat can be heard with stethoscope

End of 6th lunar mth— Fetus is 12" long, large head, skin is very wrinkled, eyelids open and close

End of 7th lunar mth— Fetus is 14" long, thin and scrawny, reddish skin, if born poor chance of survival

End of 8th lunar mth— Fetus is 16" long, hair on head more abundant, thin and wrinkled, if born there is a good chance of survival

DOCTOR'S OFFICE

End of 9th lunar mth— Fetus is 18" long, fat develops underskin giving plumper look, if born excellent chance of survival

10 lunar mth—Fetus is 20" long, fullterm 5½ to 11 lbs. average wt.

Contraception-Abortion Lifeline

Glenn E. Richardson is in the department of health and physical education at Texas A&M University, College Station, Texas 77843.

When using values clarification techniques, health educators often tend to overlook valuable teaching opportunities within the structure of the value clarifying experience. The valuing experience helps keep students' attention while incorporating facts in an interesting manner. A technique that deals with the sensitive issues of abortion and contraception and yet integrates both teaching and valuing is what I call the contraception-abortion life line. The technique can be adapted to a 20-minute period or continued for several hours of discussion depending on age group, objectives of the unit, and facilitator skills.

Method

On the chalk board or on a large piece of paper, the instructor first draws a life-line with some key points labeled.

A values question is then asked, "When does life begin?" Students respond independently until all who want to respond, do. An "L" for life is placed on the continuum for each voluntary response.

Once the students have privately or openly contemplated where life begins, a cognitive discussion of contraception and abortion methods can ensue. For each method of contraception discussed, put a mark on the continuum above the life line. The decision of where to place the contraceptive method depends on the action of the contraceptive method.

For example, the condom, foams, jellies, and diaphragm could be placed at a point between 2 and 3 because they prevent the sperm from reaching the egg. The IUD would be placed between 4 and 5 because the IUD prevents implantation of the fertilized egg. Vasectomies would be placed between 1 and 2 since the sperm is never deposited. This allows for an interesting discussion of the contraceptive techniques and can be explained in conjunction with the use of contraceptive kits.

Following the discussion of contraceptive techniques, abortion techniques can be discussed and the periods of most appropriate use be placed on the lifeline. For example, D & C and suction techniques cover points 5 through 10. Induced labor with saline solution could cover points 10 through 12.

After the cognitive portion of the technique is finished, then the valuing questions begin. Questions such as the following can be used:

1. Which, if any, of the contraceptive methods is acceptable to you intellectually? Spiritually? Emotionally? Socially? For what reasons?

2. Which, if any, of the abortion methods is acceptable to you intellectually? Spiritually? Emotionally? Socially? For what reasons?

The final question in the technique is one that will reinforce personal values or promote the examination of personal values in a way that personal affective and cognitive value dissonance will be avoided or clarified. The question is: Is the mark where you believe life begins on the right or left of your personally accepted contraceptive or abortive methods? If the life mark is on the right of the acceptable contraceptive and abortive techniques, then the preventive action of the methods occurs before life begins and no dissonance related to terminating life should be experienced. But if the life mark is on the left of the methods, then in the perception of the individual, the method takes action after life has begun and potentially could be the source of mental and emotional guilt feelings if the methods are used.

The final question can lead to a discussion of how to find peace of mind when using contraceptive methods, that is, using appropriate methods (if any) which conform to one's own values. If students are unsure when life begins, as many are, then the technique will probably stimulate some pondering. It can also lead to a discussion of the ease of modifying behaviors (use or non-use of contraceptive methods) versus the facility of changing values.

Other questions can be developed to relate the lifeline to other values, e.g., questions regarding spontaneous abortion and life, therapeutic abortion and values, and decisions to abort, keep the child, or give it up for adoption.

The abortion-contraception lifeline, a confluent education technique, places a traditional discussion of contraception and abortion methods within a valuing framework. The technique has been used many times in university classes and has provided a stimulating, clarifying, and valuable experience for teacher and students.

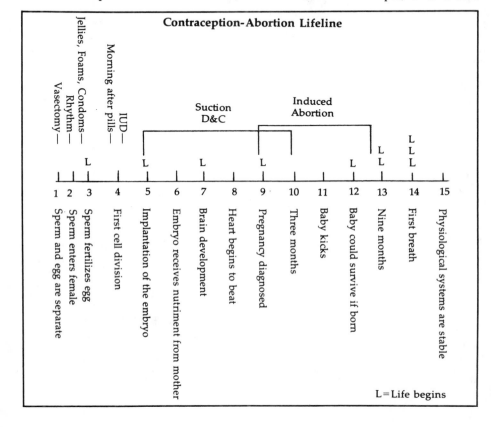

Contraception-Abortion Lifeline

Jellies, Foams, Condoms—
Rhythm—
Vasectomy—

Morning after pills—

IUD—

Suction
D&C

Induced
Abortion

L = Life begins

1 2 3 4 5 6 7 8 9 10 11 12 13 14 15

Sperm and egg are separate
Sperm enters female
Sperm fertilizes egg
First cell division
Implantation of the embryo
Embryo receives nutriment from mother
Brain development
Heart begins to beat
Pregnancy diagnosed
Three months
Baby kicks
Baby could survive if born
Nine months
First breath
Physiological systems are stable

Teaching Students About Their Future Role as Parents

JAN YOUNG is a health issues instructor in the Mankato Public Schools, Mankato, Minnesota 56001. She is a member of the AAHE Board of Directors.

Isn't it interesting, when we think of all of the time and effort that is spent in curriculum development and curricular changes, to realize that we have frequently made a complete circle to find ourselves back where we started? This appears to be more and more evident in the trend to go back to the "open school," to nongraded classrooms, and to teachers working with students of different grades and certainly different interests and talents.

In our attempts to concentrate on technical and scientific advances in knowledge, and our efforts to ensure the proper sequential development of certain basic knowledge and skills, is it possible that sometimes we overlook that which is the most obvious? Are we so concerned about what *we* think the student should know that we tend to overlook what they so desperately need for *their* future mental and social happiness?

In my 11th grade health classes, whenever I pose the question or design an activity relating to future goals, at least three-quarters of every class indicates that some day in their future they plan on being a parent. We give them instruction in many other areas and subjects, but educators neglect to spend much time on the subject of "how to be a better parent."

It is the "in thing" for many students in high school today to talk about how their parents "just don't understand" and are really not "hip" or "in tune" with what is going on. We who work with students every day see much evidence of parent-teen conflicts.

Talk about "learning opportunities"! Let's start taking advantage of these "teachable moments" in our health classes! For a perfect starter, the next time you hear any of your students make a negative remark about their parents, you can come back with the statement, "Well, I suppose they have had little or no training in how to be a parent and so perhaps it would be nice to allow them to make a few mistakes." This, or some similar statement, can get you off the ground into some very interesting "parent training" concepts.

Another interest getter is to write in large letters across the blackboard—TODAY'S LESSON: HOW TO WIN AN ARGUMENT WITH YOUR PARENTS. I can guarantee you their undivided attention!

Recently, I was among the guest speakers at a conference on "interpersonal relationships" at a local high school. A variety of topics were offered simultaneously throughout the day and students chose the five they were most interested in. My assigned topic was "human sexuality and transactional analysis," and for the first session not one student stopped by. They were attracted to the more obviously intriguing rooms labeled "vagabonding Europe," "why you shouldn't get married," and "medical aspects of abortion." Before the second session began, I put a new sign on the door that read: "How to win an argument with your parents!" For that and the remaining sessions, I had a full house, with enthusiastic students. I covered the same material that I had intended to cover, but took a different approach. We discussed many of the concepts from the book by Thomas Gordon, *Parent Effectiveness Training*, and Thomas Harris's book, *I'm OK—You're OK*. By putting myself in their place and approaching parent-teen conflicts from their view, the motivation was there—and the learning outcomes were evidenced by their comments and participation in role playing.

Many basic concepts included in a health class also relate to basic content areas in parenting.
1. *Growth and Development:* A parent who understands growth and development will be better prepared to adjust to changes in offspring.
2. *Attitudes and Habits:* A parent who is knowledgeable about the influence of the home in fostering healthy versus unhealthy attitudes will be more apt to convey positive health attitudes and habits.
3. *Communicative Skills:* A parent who is aware of common communication blocks and adept at using positive communicating skills will have a better chance of fostering and maintaining good family communication.
4. *Decision Making Skills:* Parents who allow their children to make some choices will probably have teenagers and adults who will be more responsible in making decisions that affect their health and welfare.
5. *Coping with Crisis:* Parents who understand that children learn how to cope with crisis situations will be more likely to set a better example for the children in how they as a parent meet a crisis in their family.
6. Parents' concern for their own development of maximum quality of physical, social, and mental health will hopefully develop a similar concern in their offspring.

These concepts are included in many health education programs, but those concerned with communicative skills and decision-making skills are often overlooked. Therefore the remaining part of this article will deal with methods to use these skills in teaching about parenting in a classroom.

The three main skills in parent effectiveness training that I find myself using over and over again in my health classes are:
1. *Active Listening:* this is the ability to understand what the person is "feeling" as well as saying.
2. *Use of "I Messages":* An "I message" consists of three parts:

(1) how you feel, (2) the situation or problem, and (3) the effect or reason.
3. *Who Owns the Problem:* Sometimes a conflict resolves itself when we decide whether it is really *our* problem or something we are *making* our problem. If the problem is *owned* by both parties involved, often a compromise is necessary.

Some examples of the three techniques and how they might be used by a parent, a teacher, or a teenager are given below:

SITUATION: A parent is totally frustrated by her daughter's disregard for house hours or policies established for school nights, weekends, etc.

Positive Parent Responses:
1. "You really seemed upset when I questioned you after you came home late." (active listening response)
2. "I feel bad that you came in so late since I thought we had made an agreement on weekday hours." (I message.)
3. They both own the problem. It is definitely a problem for the mother, because of her concern for daughter's ability to keep up in school. It is a problem for the daughter so long as she is a member of the family living in the same household.

By using either active listening or an "I message" or both, the parent is taking some of the pressure off and may avoid a more serious confrontation than using typical parent responses, which immediately put the person on the defensive, such as: "What is the matter with you anyway?" "When I was your age, if I came in that late I would have been campused for a month." "How do you ever expect to amount to anything? You will never be able to keep a job if you can't obey some orders."

Classroom Strategies
1. Role play family-teenage conflicts in groups or partners.
2. Practice using "I messages" in response to certain situations with a partner.
3. Conduct small group discussions about common teenage-parent conflicts and how to handle them using active listening, "I messages" and transactional analysis positions.

In role playing involving common conflicts, suggest role playing using typical responses in contrast to responses using active listening and "I messages" or problem ownership.

SITUATION I: Jim and Father have frequent arguments over use of the car. Jim feels he should be able to use the car for his dates and his father feels that he should get a job and buy his own car because he thinks Jim does not take good care of the car—leaves it in a mess and uses too much gas.

SITUATION II: Mary, an 11th grader, has a continual hassle at home over her messy room. It has created a lot of friction among the entire family and many heated arguments between Mary and her mother. Who owns this problem—Mary or her mother?

SITUATION III: Jackie has a constant battle every time she dates Jerome. She likes him and feels her parents are unfair and prejudiced because he has long hair and works in a service station. Jackie's parents want her to go to college and feel that her steady dating with Jerome will squelch this as Jerome is planning on taking a one-year mechanics course at a vocational school.

Health teachers can gain an understanding of how to use the main methods which are explained in Gordon's book on parent effectiveness training (PET). There are other general communication strategies which can and should be used, such as paraphrasing and receptive listening. Courses are offered in communications and human relations. The PET classes which are offered in many cities by certified instructors are an excellent way to better understand the principles involved. Practice helps and is really necessary to use the skills effectively and naturally in the classroom.

A common complaint of teenagers today revolves around conflicts with their parents. PET offers what is considered to be a no-lose method of solving conflicts. If you introduce these concepts to your high school students, they start to look at their own personal conflicts with their parents and by putting themselves in their parents' place they often gain much insight into how complicated the job of being a parent can be. They could, as a result of some parent training, become more responsible parents in the future.

Wayne J. Anderson, *Design For Family Living* (T. S. Denison Co., Minneapolis, Minnesota).
Cycle: An Interaction Unit Introducing the Stages of the Life Cycle (Interact, Lakeside, California).
Leotine Young, *The Fractured Family* (McGraw-Hill Book Co., St. Louis, 1973).
Aldous, Condon, Hill, Straus, Irving, and Tallman, eds., *Family Problem Solving* (Dryden Press, Inc., Hinsdale, Illinois, 1971).
Thomas A. Harris, *I'm OK, You're OK: A Practical Guide to Transactional Analysis* (Harper and Row, New York, 1973).
Herbert O. Brayer and Zella Cleary, *Valuing in the Family: A Workshop Guide for Parents* (Pennant Educational Materials, San Diego, California, 1972).
Thomas Gordon, *Parent Effectiveness Training: The Tested New Way to Raise Responsible Children* (Effectiveness Training Assoc., Pasadena, California, 1970).
Haim G. Ginott, *Between Parent and Child* (Macmillan Co., New York, 1965).

Ask the Students Themselves

A. GORDON BENNETT is supervisor of health, physical education, and recreation in the Elyria City Schools, Elyria, Ohio 44035.

In spite of a new liberation, including children, we are still Victorian in talking with our youngsters about intimate personal hygiene matters. Yet, they watch us act freely and without restraint; we drink to excess, smoke too much, take too many tranquillizers, eat too much of the wrong things, exercise too little and let our children get hung-up on drugs. Adults are still overly concerned about "hush-hush" and "hidden" subjects, and when anyone mentions sex education in the public schools, everyone panics.

Despite the antiquated fears of parents and the general public about the concept, Elyria High School students overwhelmingly confirmed that they want and need such a program in their city schools.

Students do not talk to their parents about the problem of venereal disease, for instance, but they are very much aware of it. Venereal disease is a small part of the total health education program, yet the statistics in this area of the total subject show us the weakness of our programs in the public schools.

Elyria High School, Elyria, Ohio has an enrollment of 2,734 students, tenth through twelfth grades. In November, 1,767 students went to the gym to see the film "Quarter Million Teenagers," participated in discussion, and were given names and addresses where they could be tested for VD by a health department official.

The next day, about three fourths of the student body were given some form of education on venereal disease. The facts presented were furnished by the State Board of Health and the State Board of Education. Examples of the stark and dismaying statistics furnished follow:

1. The U.S. is involved in the worst epidemic of venereal disease in history.
2. VD is second only to the common cold in the communicable disease field.
3. In Elyria alone the reported cases jumped from 20 to 60 in one year.
4. In Lorain County, Ohio—the twelfth most affected in Ohio—there was an increase of over 25%.
5. In the state of Ohio, reported cases increased over 20%.
6. Cleveland, Ohio had 73,880 new cases and is ranked 8th in the nation in venereal disease increase.
7. Ohio had 218,356 cases of gonorrhea reported.
8. In the U.S. there were *over five million* new cases of venereal disease in one year.
9. It is estimated by leading health authorities that *only 1 out of 8 cases of venereal disease is ever reported.*

After being exposed to those statistics, the Elyria High School students participated in a county-wide VD Awareness Week. They made posters, spent hours manning a booth for the Lorain City Health Department at the Midway Mall, and distributed literature contributed by the State Boards of Health and Education.

In an effort to determine. the attitude of students to health educaiton in general, and to the inclusion of such topics as venereal disease in health education, we asked about 85% of the student body to respond anonymously to questions such as the following:

Do you think health education should be put into our course of study? If so, when?

When did you first become interested and adventurous in sex?
Do you think venereal disease education should be included in a course in health education?
All the students responding felt that health should be taught K-12; the majority favored a formalized health education program beginning sometime between the fifth and ninth grade. None suggested beginning such a program as late as the eleventh or twelfth grade. As one student remarked during the discussion, "If we don't know it by then, it will be too late!" The students wanted health education to cover such topics as personal hygiene, grooming, VD, disease prevention, and dating.

In the area of VD education, our students felt free to acknowledge their need and lack of information. Adults are afraid to talk to their children about intimate physical subjects, but many refuse to allow knowledgeable professionals to do so. What kind of climate is it that will be all for permissiveness at home and in the school, but be almost obsessively opposed to giving young people necessary facts to protect them from the results of this much touted permissiveness?

With the kind of positive response of high school students demonstrated in the brief survey conducted at our high school, it appears imperative that communities begin to listen to young people and help them get the health education program they feel they want and need.

Students then shared their ideas with the class. Each question or implication offered by the students was written on the board for the entire class to see. (An overhead projector could be used.) Our list contained 26 items including questions or implications such as the following.

Gives new hope to couples who have been childless due to tubal problems.

May help in the discovery of new contraceptive methods.

If the child is not "normal," who is responsible?

Could reveal new information on the first hours and days of life.

One more step toward manipulation of life processes.

Could increase the population.

Women with tubal ligations who changed their minds and wanted to have a child may be able to become pregnant.

Opens door to surrogate mothers.

If several fertilized eggs die with IVF, is this abortion?

May help scientists find ways to prevent some genetic diseases.

Test Tube Considerations

DEBORAH A. DUNN *is assistant professor and health specialist in the Department of Physical Education for Women, Washington State University, Pullman, Washington 99164.*

The July 25, 1978 birth of Louise Brown, the first so-called test-tube baby, intensified an international debate over the ethical, legal, and societal implications of in vitro fertilization (IVF) as a means of human reproduction. With talk of cloning, surrogate motherhood, and parthenogenesis, it's possible that in the years to come, society's reproductive options may be in-

creased, thus placing additional decision making demands on individuals.

Through health education experiences, students can be aided in coming to grips with moral issues which may arise as a result of scientific advances in human reproduction. The following activity was designed to help college students identify a wide range of possible implications of IVF. The same format could be used to elicit consideration of other issues with far-reaching possibilities.

After a review of the actual procedure involved in IVF, the students were asked to recall the reactions of various individuals and groups to the announcement of the first successful IVF. How did prominent scientists and theologians react? How was it handled by the press? What did your family, friends, or acquaintances have to say about it? How did you react to the news?

Keeping these reactions to IVF in mind, the students were asked to silently list some of the questions that had been raised and some of the implications that had been identified. What legal questions have surfaced? How might it affect the family? What could it mean to science?

When all questions or implications were on the board, students wrote out the three they thought carried that most importance in the debate over this form of reproduction. Then, they placed the number 3 next to the most important question or implication, a 2 by the second most important, and a 1 next to the third most important. The papers were collected and the scores were tallied. The most commonly identified concerns were the question of responsibility should the child be deformed, the new hope given to couples who could not conceive, the fear of manipulation of life processes, and the possibility of the procedure leading to new contraceptive methods.

The followup to the exercise consisted of a discussion of why the questions and implications that were most often raised by the students were worthy of such careful thought and consideration.

Family Life

Selected Impacts of Contraception on Man and/or Society

PATRICK KIDD TOW is a graduate assistant in the Department of Health Education at Southern Illinois University, Carbondale, Illinois 62901.

This teaching strategy was designed primarily for college health survey classes, however, it could also be applied to students in the senior high school setting. This activity could follow after a unit on population growth, human sexuality, or birth control education. It involves dividing a class into separate groups to brainstorm a list of all possible impacts from the usage of contraceptive methods. The topic can be examined in view of the impact upon the individual or society as a whole. Fifteen minutes are usually allotted for this portion.

After this step has been accomplished, their next announced objective would be assigning symbols to each derived impact. These symbols (=, −, or ?) would represent respectively, whether they felt the concerned impact is desirable, undesirable, or questionable. Value judgments must be made as a group. There will be some items that are obviously controversial, therefore, it would be advisable for the classroom teacher to circulate and help facilitate the discussions when necessary. This portion of the activity usually involves about 15 minutes.

Bringing the groups back together as a class, the teacher calls upon a member from each group to share the findings on the emotional impacts of contraceptive usage. On the second round, a different member in each group presents the environmental outcomes. This process continues until all six areas of concern are brought out for classroom discussion and everyone has an opportunity to present their group consensus. This final part should take approximately 20 minutes.

Symbol Designations
+ = positive or desirable
− = negative or undesirable
? = questionable

Emotional Impacts
1. eases fear of pregnancy out of a loving relationship (+)
2.
3.

Physical Impacts
1. contraceptive devices may cause cancer (−)
2.
3.

Social Impacts
1. inlaws frown upon childless couple (−)
2.
3.

Environmental Impacts
1. human race may become extinct (?)
2.
3.

Economic Impacts
1. parents are afforded more time and money to plan family (+)
2.
3.

Religious Impacts
1. considered a violation of religious beliefs by ministers (−)
2.
3.

First Aid and Safety

A Working Model for Simulation Techniques

GLEN G. GILBERT is instructor of health education, University of North Carolina at Greensboro, Greensboro, North Carolina 27412. Much of the material for this article is from the ongoing research by the author for his doctoral dissertation at Ohio State University.

Instructors of emergency care are faced with the challenge of educating personnel to deal with complex situations that require prompt and efficient treatment. The instructor, largely because of time limitations, is often forced to rely on "one shot" coverage of the individual skills involved. Commonly such coverage is followed by a paper and pencil test in an attempt to evaluate the students' ability to apply specific skills.

This article presents an alternative method of teaching and evaluating those skills dealt with in emergency health care classes. It promotes confidence in the students' ability to employ the newly acquired skills in real life situations, presenting a variety of situations that require the application of a multiplicity of first aid skills.

The use of simulated emergency care situations is not a new idea, but this article presents several new variations on simulation design and provides a working model for those persons unfamiliar with simulation techniques.

Simulated situations can be an asset to any emergency care program for the following reasons:

1. They provide examples of real life emergency care situations.

2. They provide practical applications of skills covered in the classroom.

3. They provide practice in the analysis and evaluation of emergency situations without possible injury resulting from judgment errors.

4. They provide an alternate teaching strategy for the instructor.

5. They provide a possible evaluation technique for instructors.

6. They provide students with practice in performing skills under stress and thereby should increase self-confidence.

Simulations can become an integral part of an emergency care instructional program from the onset. They can be used in a variety of ways, some of which are outlined below:

1. They can be used as a direct communication strategy by presenting the situation and the correct performance of first aid procedures by the instructor or the student.

2. They can serve as an instructor-student interaction strategy by presenting the situation and jointly (instructor and class) analyzing the proper course of action and reasoning.

3. They can be a group activity with several people working out a course of action and then undertaking it. This might be better in more complicated situations.

4. They can function as an independent student activity by setting up an area where students come in and perform skills in varied situations.

You may wish to devise your own simulation situations or ask your students to make them up for you, in which case each student should design one situation complete with symptoms and procedures. A file of such student situations can be collected and made available to students for review.

The Simulation Model: Scenario

The student selected to perform as a first aider selects a card, reads the number, and leaves the room.[1] While he is out of the room the situation numbered is set up. Other students are employed as victims with symptom tags, medical alert tags, or whatever is appropriate for the situation, placed on their person. These tags are put at the site of the simulated injury or symptom. The materials which are available to the first aider are placed in the area designated as the situation area.

The student re-enters the room upon notification and reads the card out loud to the class (he is allowed to keep it during the situation). He then examines the situation, makes a judgment based upon the symptom tags, and other information provided, and then performs the proper first aid procedures. The instructor rates the student's performance using a predesigned form.

The more realistic a situation, the better it is as a learning device. There are simulation kits available that include simulated injuries and simulated bleeding which can be used, but they require a much larger amount of time and the cost is often high. The major

---

[1]Selection of situation cards should be accomplished by shuffling and the taking of the top card each time or some other method at the discretion of the instructor. However, it is advised that a random device be employed so that students will not feel their situation was predetermined at the will of the instructor.

advantage of the system described here is that it is relatively fast and inexpensive while providing a good deal of realism.

You may wish to add certain realistic touches such as turning out the lights to simulate night time, adding more props, or even having victims chew cookies and simulate vomiting. The extent to which you carry this is limited only by your imagination.

Critique

Following the completion of situations it is recommended that a critique be held, explaining the proper procedures and clearing up any questions. This can be done after each situation, at the close of each session, or at the end of all the situations depending on the instructor's time schedule and wishes. Copies of the rating form may be distributed and used by fellow students during the performance, for comparison and to reinforce learning. They can also be collected by the instructor to aid him in his rating.

Another technique is to employ overhead projections (showing correct procedures) during the situation, but in such a manner that the participating first aider cannot see them. Flashing the projection immediately after completion of a situation is a technique which also saves class time that normally would be taken reviewing each different situation at a later time.

In the majority of situations several alternate first aid procedures are possible and appropriate. The design of evaluation forms should take this into consideration. Evaluation should be based only on the results of the first aid and not the appearance of any special bandage the instructor had in mind. The intention is to help save lives, not win a neatness contest. However, effective bandages are most often neatly applied.

Preparation for the Instructor

The instructor should develop and review the situations to be sure he understands the correct procedures and has all the proper materials necessary. Tags and other materials should be kept in separate envelopes and numbered for easy access. Masking tape can serve to hold tags in place. Assistants should be recruited and trained to ensure that the situations will be set up rapidly.

The instructor should review all instructions with participants and should present a sample situation.

The makeup of each class determines the situations. First aid for housewives should emphasize more household accidents and first aid for firemen should emphasize burns, smoke inhalation, and so on.

Careful selection of victims is necessary. Some situations require little acting ability (e.g. an unconscious victim), but others require a great deal of showmanship to be effective (e.g., drug freakout). Try to involve everyone at least once as a victim or bystander. You may wish to employ "professional" victims to ensure that the simulations will be well done.

SAMPLE EVALUATION FORM
TRANSFER-BREATHING-BLEEDING

Circle the appropriate number and total at the bottom. Values should be assigned according to the importance of each skill.

	YES Well Done	YES Adequate	NO
1. Was the victim examined quickly for all possible injuries?	3-2	1	0
2. Was the victim quickly removed from imminent danger by an appropriate method? *Note—lack of speed would be a deduction here.	6-5-4	3-2-1	0
3. Was victim given proper mouth-to-mouth artificial respiration until victim revives? 　A. Clear Obstructions (1) 　B. Proper head tilt (2) 　C. Timing (1) 　D. Dealing with difficulties (1) *Note—in some cases mouth-to-nose, mouth-to-stoma or a manual method may be required.	5-4	3-2-1	0
4. Was victim given proper care for mild bleeding? 　A. Direct pressure and elevation (1) 　B. Proper bandage (2)	3-2	1	0
5. Was victim given verbal encouragement? *Note—just saying you will be OK isn't very good verbal encouragement.	2	1	0
6. Was victim treated for shock? *Note—remember shock treatment varies.	2	1	0
7. Was proper additional/ professional aid called for?	2	1	0

Add _____ +2 _____

Deductions _____

Total_____

Possible___ 25 _____

Comments:
　—Additions can be used to equalize situations so they all have the same point values.
　—Deductions include improper order such as treating a fracture before life threatening bleeding.

SAMPLE SITUATION

> Situation:
>   Your brother is playing in the garage when you hear an explosion. There is smoke in the air and the roof appears in danger of collapsing.
> Where:
>   Your home.
> Miscellaneous Information:
>   No one else is home.

Above is the card that is given to the first aider. The information below is not seen by the first aider. It gives the directions for the conduct of the simulation.
Position of victim:
    Face down.
Special Instructions for Victim:
    Remain unconscious until signaled by instructor.
Special Instructions for bystanders:
    No bystanders present.
Supplied Materials:
1. Home materials box (a box containing those first aid supplies generally found in the home.)
Tags:
1. No air going in or out (1) chest
2. Blue skin (1) face
3. Mild bleeding (1) right forearm

PARTICIPANTS INSTRUCTIONS

1. You must treat this *like a real life situation.* Nothing will be assumed—you must do all that you would in a real life situation. To receive credit for any procedure it must be accomplished completely. The only exception to this is procedures that cannot be done in the classroom such as making a phone call.

2. You may use only material *provided* in the testing area.
3. You may *not* use any notes or cards other than those provided.
4. For assistance you may use only those people provided and *you must give* explicit directions for any aid they administer. No undirected assistance or information is to be given by other students or victims.
5. *Time will be an important factor in life threatening situations.* A reasonable time will be allowed for less severe injuries, but do not waste time. (After having used a situation several times an instructor will have an idea of how long it should take to complete and may wish to set a time limit.)

SIMULATION TAGS

Simulation tags which have symptoms written on them are constructed for each situation and attached to victims by masking tape. They are coded by color—red for bleeding, blue for breathing difficulties and cold, green and yellow for miscellaneous symptoms.

Their size is appropriate for the symptom. This means that symptoms that would be obvious such as severe bleeding, have a large tag and clear fluid from the ear, are relatively small. No attempt is made to hide tags any more than in real situations. The objective is not to trick anyone, but rather to ensure a thorough examination.

Burns are listed by degrees for easy identification of proper first aid treatment. Bleeding tags are marked mild, moderate, or severe.

In appropriate situations medical alert tags and cards plus medications are supplied to further aid the first aider in diagnosis. Medications are given in several cases to ensure understanding of the Red Cross position on providing or giving medication. Names on medications and cards should be uni-sex (i.e., Pat) so that male or female victims fit into all situations.

First Aid and Safety

Breaking the Accident Chain

Richard T. Mackey is in the Department of Health and Physical Education at Miami University, Oxford, Ohio 45056.

"Accidents don't just happen, they are caused." It's a simple straightforward statement, but how tough it is to convince people of its validity.

An "accident chain" is an effective instructional device for helping individuals analyze the causes of many types of accidents. It can be used in school health instruction or in an industrial setting. Here's how it works.

The "accident chain" consists of a 2 ×4 length of wood with six, 2 ×2 inch pieces resting on one-half inch dowels cut lengthwise. The dowels are glued to the 2 × 4s. Grooves are cut in the 2 × 2s so they rest on the dowels. The six upright pieces contain chain words and are placed six inches apart so that when any one is removed the chain action will be interrupted when the pieces are toppled. The removal of one word represents the removal of one factor which leads to an accident. Thus the accident

chain will not be activated and symbolically the accident will not have occurred.

The first upright represents environmental factors such as: crowding, doors, drinking fountain, floors, lighting, no handrails or weather. The second represents human factors such as: active game, fatigue, horseplay, lack of training or experience, running, violation of rules. Next comes the agent which includes: animal or insect, electricity, fire, gases, liquids, recreational equipment, pencil, student, or vehicle. The trigger is the actual incident which results in the accident. The slipping of the car tires on the pavement, the bat flying out of the student's hands, the toe of the person's foot catching on the stairstep, the rug slipping on the floor, are all examples of

the trigger. There are conditions when all the elements leading to an accident are present but nothing triggers it. There must be a trigger for an accident to occur, but if the other factors are changed or eliminated the trigger will not be activated.

In analyzing the accidents ask your students questions such as: What were the environmental factors? How could the conditions been changed to prevent the accident? What was the agent? What was the trigger? How could the situation been changed to avoid activating the trigger?

All accidents can be analyzed with the accident chain model. Why not add it to your instructional devices. Figures 1 and 2 show the accident chain before and after being activated.

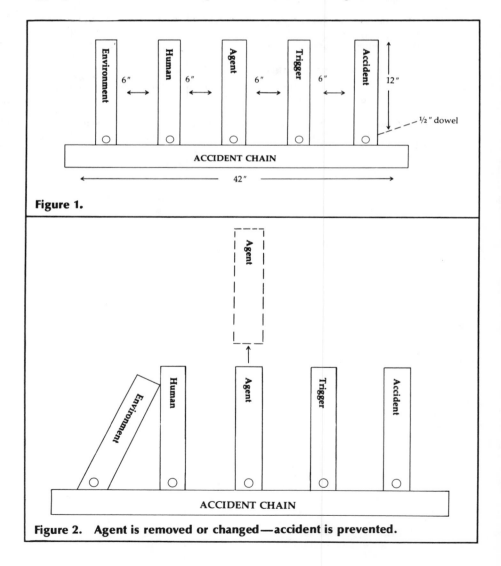

Figure 1.

Figure 2. Agent is removed or changed—accident is prevented.

CPR Drilling

MARK KITTLESON is an instructor in the Health Education Department at Youngstown State University, Youngstown, Ohio 44503. He is currently certified as an instructor-trainer in CPR by the American Heart Association.

Cardiopulmonary resuscitation (CPR) has been making a lot of headlines lately. Several states have now mandated CPR instruction to all high school students before they are allowed to graduate. Many people are turning to the health educator to provide this CPR training. Through the help of the American Heart Association many health educators are receiving this training to teach such courses. Unfortunately, most schools cannot provide the necessary equipment to effectively teach a CPR course. This article discusses problems the CPR instructor will encounter and possible solutions to them.

Problems

There are several problems that health educators face when teaching CPR in almost every learning situation—high school, community college, university, community.

1. Size of Class—It is common to have a great number of students enrolled in first aid or CPR classes, which makes learning difficult. Many institutions, such as the University of Maine at Farmington, limit class size. A large group limits individual help and many students may feel neglected. Other universities, such as Mankato State University, have access to paramedic students who are also instructors. This does alleviate the problem somewhat.

2. Time—Invariably, a few students cannot achieve the certification because the manikins must be returned at a certain date. If you are in a high school or college that does not own its own manikins, you must reserve them from institutions (e.g. American Heart Association, Red Cross, hospitals, ambulance crews) and it might take several weeks before they are available.

Much time is wasted during the actual class period. Only two people can work on a manikin at a time, thus several students must sit around and wait. Telling students to work with one another in-

dependently on a procedure usually does not work. Most students need more structured instruction.

3. Lack of Manikins—Many schools and universities cannot afford manikins. For those who can, few have the proper number to effectively teach CPR (a 6–1 ratio is recommended by the American Heart Association).

4. Areas of Certification—The American Heart Association requires that students master four areas before they are certified—obstructed airway, infant resuscitation, single and two person rescue. It seems almost impossible for one instructor to teach all those areas to a large group of students, but it can be done. All it takes is a little imagination, a little "army regimentation," and a strong voice.

5. Limitations of Manikins—Although the recording manikins are well constructed, they do lack the human touch in several areas. It is important that students work on the following areas on a real human.

(1) The nostrils on the doll need to be tough to stand the wear and tear, which makes them more difficult to pinch than a human nose.
(2) The doll's neck is more rigid than a human's, so students need to practice opening the airway on a real human. By doing so they find the head tilts much easier.
(3) Palpating the pulse is one of the most important techniques. CPR done on a person with a beating heart could result in serious damage. The instructor must emphasize the importance of taking at least 10 seconds to find the pulse. Students should practice taking a pulse on a live person to know what that pulse feels like, where to find it, and how hard to press.
(4) Finding the xiphoid on the manikins is not as effective. Everybody has a different placement for the xiphoid, thus it is important that the students have the opportunity to find xiphoids on several other humans. This is an area of concern because if the xiphoid is pressed on, it will break off and cause internal bleeding.
(5) When you are working on a human, you need to be gentle. When working with a manikin, this gentleness seems to diminish after a few hours. The shake and shout procedure, which is the first step in CPR, can be misinterpreted as a "slugfest" with the victim. Rescuers get a feeling of how hard to shake if they work on a real human. Students learn to gently open the airway when working with a real subject. It is possible when working with a manikin to throw the airway open abruptly, which could be hazardous to the victim.

Class Management

A large class can be successfully managed. First concentrate on procedure; manikins are not needed. Once the procedure is in student memory, learning proper compression depth and ventilation will come fairly quickly with practice on a manikin.

The following procedure works best for me. Other instructors must adapt it to their needs.

Line students up in the hallway in groups of threes. The victims lie on the floor or on several blankets with their heads in the same direction. One student is the observer and stands at the head of the victim. Because of the large number of students it is difficult for the instructor to observe every student. The observer can spot any major mistakes. The third student is the rescuer. All rescuers should kneel on the same side of the victim to prevent confusion when giving instructions; when you say right hand you mean everybody's right hand.

Start with the shake and shout and then opening the airway. Go through the entire procedure until you feel the students have mastered the skill. Make sure students switch around to experience all three roles.

There are several major areas that need repeated work.

1. Moving from chest to mouth and back to the chest in five seconds. This teaches the student to move quickly to the mouth and get back to the chest to find proper hand position. You can drill students—"Find hand position, go to mouth and ventilate; find landmark and hand position, go to mouth and ventilate, etc." Give the students five seconds to ventilate before instructing them to find the landmarks. Drilling for only two minutes can give them the feel for moving quickly.

2. Counting properly for efficient output. Have the student put hands in position on the chest and *without* compression, count at the right rate, then move to the head and ventilate, and go back to the chest. Students can count together or individually. Use a stop watch to see if the students are counting at the proper rate.

3. Switching with a second rescuer. The major problem in the two person rescue is the switch. Locate one rescuer at the head and the second at the chest. The instructor should do the counting and tell the rescuers when to switch. You can see any mixups, which there will be the first few times. Keep this procedure going until you feel the students have mastered this procedure.

4. Finding the xiphoid. A simple drilling technique is to have the students find the landmark (xiphoid), then take their hands off the chest. Keep drilling the students by giving only two seconds to find the landmark and then having them drop their hands.

These drills allow the instructor to teach the students the basic procedure before they even have a chance to get on the manikin. This will reduce needless work on the manikins and reduce idle time; every person is involved. The observer notes whether or not the rescuer is doing the procedure properly, and the victim can inform the rescuer if the hand position is incorrect. Doing this procedure for two hours will drill the proper procedure into the students. Students can concentrate on perfecting the proper compression depth and ventilation rate when they get on the manikin, instead of wasting time learning the procedure on the manikins.

Alternatives to Manikins

If you have a large class and lack enough manikins, you can still give students a simulated compression and ventilation activity. Collect liquid soap bottles and rinse them out. Fill the bottles about three-quarters full with water and reseal the caps. Students should use proper hand position on the bottle and compress. This gives a pretty good idea of compression. Be prepared for occasional leaks.

For ventilation simulation, collect old fabric softener or similar bottles and rinse them out thoroughly. Attach a large balloon to the opening. With a knife, make a small slice in the middle of the bottle and insert the opening of a small balloon in it. Make a larger hole (to stimulate a mouth) below the small balloon. What you have basically is a head and lung. Blowing into the mouth will inflate both balloons; however, in CPR you pinch the nostrils, and thus in this simulation you pinch the smaller balloon. This gives a pretty good idea of how much effort is needed to ventilate a real human. Naturally, these two simulations cannot match a manikin or a human, but they are simple, cheap techniques to teach the general principles of CPR.

Mental Health

On The Level
A New TV Series for and about Teenagers

Gus T. Dalis is a consultant in health education and teaching strategies in the office of the Los Angeles County Superintendent of Schools.

The concluding scene is the high school yearbook office. Alice's boyfriend, Jerry enters . . .

> *Alice, I should have known you'd be here. Back at the scene of the crime . . . Listen, do you know what's going on?*
>
> *'Course I know, did you think I didn't see Gail before I left the table?*
>
> *So go and deal with her, will ya?*
>
> *Leave me alone, Jerry!*
>
> *But you started the whole blasted war!*
>
> *It's none of your business. Why don't you just get out of here!*
>
> *Hey, look who's getting mad. Go shout like that at Gail!*
>
> *Don't you tell me what to do! And get something straight, I don't like to fight with people, I can't stand up to anybody and I'm tired of you rubbing my face into it all of the time!*

Alice is startled by the sudden opening of the door. It's Gail . . .

> *Uh, hi Alice.*
>
> *Gail! What do you want?*
>
> *I wanted to talk to you . . . can I come in? Come on . . . let me in.*
>
> *Alright . . . come on in . . . we have a lot to talk about.*

The door closes, the screen goes black and the credits appear. The end? Not really. It is really a beginning. By using a group setting and surrounding it with relevant discussion questions and activities, teachers can use dramatizations such as this one about conflict to get at some of the gut-level issues affecting teenagers.

On The Level Series

The above scene is from a program in *On The Level*, a classroom video series for fourteen-to-seventeen year olds that is being broadcast during the school day by many PBS stations. This series consists of twelve 15-minute programs, each of which dramatizes a problem in the lives of this age group. Program topics include: Developing self-concept, accepting feelings, facing conflict, thinking,

The problem here is that Sam doesn't want to be a baker, even though he's taken over the family bakery for his ailing father. The scene is from On the Level, *a new classroom video series for teenagers that focuses on personal and social growth.*

Tyrone, a would-be jazz artist, searches for his identity in "Who Am I?" a program about self-concept that is part of On the Level.

changing family relationships, alone vs. lonely, friendship, coping with stress, career aspirations, peer group membership, prejudice, and love.

Through program viewing along with pre- and post-viewing discussion and activity, students are provided the opportunity to explore the series topics. It is intended that this exploration will yield certain personal and social growth outcomes for students. These outcomes include increased:

- Awareness of the interaction of emotional and physical health;

- Skill in identifying and analyzing the interplay between feelings and outward behavior;

- Understanding of causes of emotional stress and ability to cope constructively with such stress;

- Understanding of their relations with peers, non-parental adults, parents, and younger children.

Accompanying the video series is a Leader's/Teacher's Guide. Included in this guide for each of the 12 video dramatizations is a program summary, background information about the program topic, student outcomes, before-and-after-viewing-the-program questions and activities, and reproducible activity sheets. Each *On The Level* video program has been adapted in an audio format. Unlike the video programs which are open-ended, each audio program gives several alternate endings. Creative use of this audio component should help adolescents discover that there are a variety of different ways to deal with a given issue. A student activity book is also available. It serves as a personal guide to help teenagers explore the life issues dealt with in *On The Level*. The guide includes self quizzes, readings on the topics, and activities to encourage thinking, writing and doing. Students can use the guide for independent study or for an accompaniment to the *On The Level* video or audio series.

Series Development

The *On The Level* series was produced by the Agency for Instructional Television (AIT), a nonprofit American-Canadian agency, in conjunction with a consortium of 32 state and provincial education agencies. Additional funding support came from the Corporation for Public Broadcasting, Exxon Corporation, General Mills, the George Gund Foundation and Union Carbide.

The series is designed to promote the personal and social growth of youngsters fourteen-to-seventeen years old. The series developers define personal and social growth as *a process that fosters possession of skills, information, and attributes needed to shape life events and make constructive and maturing responses in those events. In this context, life events are changes in physical make-up, intellectual development, personal feelings, or changes in relations with others or with the physical environment.*[1]

132

Planning for the series began in 1977. Using a prospectus published in 1978, AIT staff and consortium representatives sharply defined the series goals in 1979. The project design team developed, in the fall of that year, twelve program topics, each considered relevant to the personal and social growth of high school age youngsters.

In order to validate the program topics and student outcomes, secondary school teachers and other professionals likely to use the series were interviewed in groups and asked to complete a take-home questionnaire. They found the topics in personal and social growth to be familiar and important. There was a general feeling that many of these topics are now included in a variety of curriculum areas, that the intensity and manner in which they are covered varies, and that some topics are distinctly more difficult to teach than others. In addition, the teachers thought that the series would be an important tool for engaging teachers and students in discussions of these relevant issues.

From here the series was put into production. Extensive evaluation was conducted with 4,000 teenagers and their teachers during production. The programs provided the catalyst for teenagers to discuss issues of importance to them. Teenagers reacted sometimes strongly, sometimes timidly, but almost always with the acknowledgement that they were concerned about the issues and appreciated the opportunity to talk about them.

On the basis of student as well as teacher reactions many changes were made in the treatment and scripts. Revisions included: character and plot alterations to make the characters and situations more realistic and relevant to teenagers; and dialogue changes to enhance the program's message and make the programs more comprehensible.

Vehicle for Affective Education

Through experience AIT has found that video programming, when properly shaped, can be useful in enhancing the affective curriculum in school settings. Such series as *Ripples* and *Inside/Out* for the elementary school level and *Self Incorporated* for the junior high level represent efforts to assist teachers in dealing with affective issues in the area of personal growth and development. With the completion of the *On The Level* series AIT has achieved a K–12 affective education program in the area of health education.

The programs for all these AIT series are particularly helpful in facilitating affective learnings. That is, when properly used they are useful in helping students explore their own beliefs, opinions, and likes and dislikes.

Effective Use of the Series

Essentially, proper use of the *On The Level* series involves (1) selection of appropriate questions and activities to precede and follow the program, and (2) the establishment of psychological freedom in the classroom or group setting.

The Leader's/Teacher's Guide contains a pool of questions and activities useful in "squeezing health education affective juice" out of the series. For example, in using the program "Face to Face," which centers around the conflict between Alice and Gail, one of the teachers participating in evaluation of that program selected the following from the Guide:

Before the Program
- Get a group agreement on the definition of conflict. Discuss some of the factors that help to determine the severity of conflict.
- In small groups, make a list of the positive things that can result from conflict. The negative things.

After the Program
- Ask students to respond to the following questions: What were the conflicts in Alice's life? Did any of these conflicts have an effect on Alice's physical and emotional health? If so, how?
- Have each person write an ending to the program's story line. (What happened when Gail and Alice confronted each other?) Discuss the different endings.
- Complete the reproducible activity "How Do You Handle Conflict?" located in the back of the guidebook (this is an instrument useful in determining ways people handle conflict).
- Invite students to discuss the following question: How do you feel about facing conflict?

The most critical element in the successful use of *On The Level* is the teacher. That is, what the teacher does and does not do as he or she *interacts* with teenagers will determine the degree of success or failure in using the series. In addition to utilizing relevant questions and activities, the teacher needs to create a classroom environment that allows free, open and responsible discussion. Such a psychologically free environment should allow diversity without the fear

of recriminations from classmates or the teacher.

To establish such an environment it is helpful for the teacher to set discussion ground rules.[2] For example, "In our discussion today let's have one person speak at a time. Remember it's OK to disagree but don't be disagreeable when you do so. Also, no put downs." As the discussion unfolds the teacher's role is to maintain the ground rules and to refrain from judging students' ideas directly or indirectly.

It was through such a teacher-established classroom environment after viewing the program on conflict that one student reported that she did not feel alone. The student communicated relief in not being "weird" because through discussion she discovered she was not the only one afraid of dealing with conflict. Somehow there seems to be a sense of security in knowing that one's peers have similar anxieties, fears, and joys. This sense of security can come to thousands of high school students if appropriate affective teaching materials as well as teaching behaviors are carefully utilized.

Perhaps the power of the *On The Level* series became most apparent when students responded with disappointment and frustration at the lack of "real" program endings. After viewing the programs students often responded with *What happened to the rest of it? When is the rest of it going to be on TV? I want to see what happens.*

Yet it was this frustration which seemed to be a viable starting point for the exploration of ideas and opinions relative to growth and development. And that is what this series is all about—providing a catalyst for the exploration of life issues relevant to high school students.

---

[1]Agency for Instructional Television. *Education for personal and social growth of secondary school students.* Bloomington, Indiana: Agency for Instructional Television, 1978.

[2]Agency for Instructional Television. *Research Report 70—Secondary health project: concepts review.* Bloomington, Indiana: Agency for Instructional Television, 1980.

[3]Dalis, Gus T. and Strasser, Ben. B. *Teaching strategies for values awareness and decision making in health education.* Thorofare, New Jersey: Charles B. Slack, Inc., 1977.

Anyone wishing further information about local availability of "On the Level" may contact: AIT, Box A, Bloomington, Indiana 47402, (812) 339-2203.

Perceptions of Me

JERROLD S. GREENBERG is coordinator of health education, State University of New York at Buffalo, Buffalo, New York 14214. He serves as contributing editor for this SHR department, which is designed to be of particular usefulness to the classroom teacher at all levels.

Though realizing the degree of immodesty of which I can be accused, let me risk stating that the most interesting topic to me is me. Further, the most interesting topic to you is probably you. That's nothing startling. We all are interested in ourselves. Realizing this phenomenon, educators recommend that learnings in school be related to the life experiences of the learner. It then seems to follow that with the learner himself the topic of study, the efficiency and effectiveness of the learning process would be maximized.

The question of the appropriateness of oneself as a topic for study within a school setting, however, remains. Since one behaves on how one perceives reality rather than upon reality itself, one's perceptions of oneself will determine many health related behaviors. For example, one

possessing a positive self-concept might be expected to walk tall (upright) while one with a negative self-concept might walk slumped over to physically indicate "lowliness"; or one with a positive sense of sexual self-esteem might be outgoing and pleasant, whereas one with a negative feeling about oneself sexually might behave in a shy, withdrawn manner.

Based upon the importance of perceptions of oneself, and, in addition, how others perceive one (since they will behave toward others based upon their perceptions of them) activities should be developed and conducted with students to help them to:

1. More realistically perceive themselves and others.
2. Explore the relationship between their perceptions and how they act.
3. Make whatever adjustments they deem necessary to become what they want to be. Presented in this article are examples of such learning activities.

Sentence Completions

Unfinished sentences which require the student to react by completing them, allow for self-inquiry of a kind to which people are not accustomed. Examples of such questions indicate the breadth of possibilities and range of topics which can be explored with this instructional strategy.

1. I often _____
2. I seldom _____
3. I'm bored when _____
4. I love to _____
5. Other children _____
6. I will _____
7. I must _____
8. I am very _____
9. I wish I could _____
10. My friends are _____
11. My parents _____
12. I wish _____
13. I feel _____
14. I'm happy when _____
15. My body _____

Whereas the completion of these sentences requires the student to think about himself, processing the responses in small groups allows

students to explore other childrens' perceptions of themselves. It is hoped that surprises about certain responses will help children be more accepting of others and better understand themselves. If the class trusts the teacher sufficiently, the reading of the responses by the teacher might also aid the teacher to better plan instruction which pertains to the needs of the students.

Discussion Questions

Using questions to stimulate group discussions is not a recent educational innovation, but the types of questions suggested for use here differ from those employed elsewhere.

1. What is the one thing that scares you the most?
2. When are you most hurt?
3. What is the very first thing that you remember?
4. What is the saddest thing that has ever happened to you?
5. What is the best thing that has ever happened to you?
6. What do you dislike most about school?
7. What don't you like about yourself?
8. What do you like most about yourself?
9. What would you rather have: wealth, intelligence, or physical attractiveness?
10. Who is the most influential person in your life?
11. What do you wish?
12. How can you be happy?
13. What do you love to do the most?
14. What was the strongest feeling you had last week (anger, joy, grief, etc. . . .) and what caused that feeling?
15. What is something you can tell us now that you wouldn't have felt comfortable telling us before?

Each group should be reminded that there are no right or wrong answers to such questions and, therefore, they should expect each person to respond differently. The group members' role should be to ask questions of the respondent which will help the group to better understand the response, rather than to attempt to get the group to agree on what would be the "best" answer. As a result of this exercise, it is anticipated that each student will have a more accurate picture of both himself and his classmates than prior to the exercise.

Question Sociogram

An activity which can be used to aid students to see themselves as others see them is the Question Sociogram. Unlike a regular sociogram which asks children to list a number of people they would like to attend a movie with, etc., the Question Sociogram asks children to place the name of the person in the class *most likely* to fit the description implicit in the question. Examples of questions which can be used will help to clarify this technique:

_____ 1) Who most likely is afraid of mice?
_____ 2) Who most likely cannot resist eating a donut?
_____ 3) Who wakes up often with nightmares?
_____ 4) Who loves cowboy movies?
_____ 5) Who loves romantic movies?
_____ 6) Who most wants a lot of money?
_____ 7) Who watches a lot of television?
_____ 8) Who most likely will be a scientist?
_____ 9) Who will be a politician?
_____ 10) Who will make the best mother or father?
_____ 11) Who will never get married?
_____ 12) Who will never use drugs?
_____ 13) Who is most likely to cheat on an exam?
_____ 14) Who will be the most thoughtful lover?
_____ 15) Who will be a talking liberal who won't do anything?
_____ 16) Who will insist on a small wedding?
_____ 17) Who would be the best teacher?
_____ 18) Who is apt to do anonymous favors for people?
_____ 19) Who will always be physically attractive?
_____ 20) Who would make the best friend?

To the left of each number, students are required to place the name of one student in their group or class. Only one name can be written on the blank line and each blank line *must* have a name on it. After the responses have been made each child can ask each other child which descriptions he most fits, thereby acquiring others' perceptions of himself. To better know oneself is the first step in improving oneself.

Intimacy Questions

Once trust has been developed in a class or group of children, questions of a more intimate nature can be explored. Best discussed in pairs to provide a close relationship, some of the following questions can be employed by a teacher willing to take risks to provide meaningful educational experiences:

1. What do you feel most ashamed of in your past?
2. What have you deliberately lied about? Why?
3. When do you hurt people?
4. What turns you on the most?
5. Do you have any health problems? What are they?
6. What are your least attractive features?
7. Do you believe in God? Organized religion?
8. Are your parents happily married? Why? Why not?
9. How do you feel when you love?
10. What makes you swear?
11. What do you think about homosexuals?
12. Do you like yourself? Why? Why not?
13. What was your greatest failure? Greatest success?

14. Who would you be if you could be anyone else that you wanted?

These questions develop greater closeness between two people who are honest and trusting to begin with, and likewise can develop greater distance between two people who feel threatened by such openness. It is important, therefore, to employ this activity only with a group that has matured and can take advantage of such an opportunity to mature further.

Enhancing Positive Self-Concept Through Creativity in the Classroom

Barbara Beier is on the academic staff in the health education department at the University of Wisconsin, La Crosse, 54601.

I am convinced that one of the major challenges to teachers and other group leaders is the creation of a self-enhancing learning environment. Some special people seem to do this quite naturally out of their own authentic being and their commitment to others. Most of us, however, benefit from suggestions or training in allowing our creative potentials to enhance a positive, humanistic environment in the classroom.

A workshop, "Creative Teaching Methods in Health," offered by the University of Wisconsin - La Crosse Division of University Outreach, allowed the creative process to surface in me. As a young health director I was quite concerned with dispensing cognitive material to my students, but I have begun to understand that young people need more than subject matter. I like to think, now, that I teach the students, not just the subject.

Creative methods for teaching health education can be written, published in books, and distributed nationwide, but these ideas are only tools. Their use depends on you. Your use of ideas to foster positive selfconcept will depend upon your own selfesteem. As John Vasconcellos states,

"Only if you are truly into your own being, possess and value yourself, feel comfortable with and good about yourself, believe in and live your right to be yourself—will you truly enhance selfesteem in those young human beings whose selfesteem, whose lives, are touched by you." [1]

Research literature is filled with reports indicating that cognitive learning increases when selfconcept increases. [2] Following is a series of creative teaching methods compiled to foster a positive selfconcept in students of health education.

Activity #1: Sharing Bags

Grade level: 10th grade

Materials needed: any size paper bag for each student, pictures, fabric, decorative findings, scissors, paste

Background information: In many classes students never have an opportunity to get acquainted with their classmates. All of us share a need for meaningful interpersonal relationships. However, many times creating a classroom environment conducive to positive interaction is awkward and difficult for teachers. This activity could be a good starting point for teachers who seek to facilitate growth in students' potential for interpersonal relationships.

Objective: The student will have the opportunity to recognize meaningful information about themselves which can be shared with classmates.

Procedure:

1. Distribute paper bags, one to each student.

2. Instruct students to select from the fabric, pictures, and decorations.

3. Illustrate on the outside of the bag how they think *other people* see them.

4. On the inside of the bag, have students illustrate how they *see themselves*—how they really are.

5. Upon completion, the bags may be shared with the entire class, with a small group or with a partner.

Follow-up questions:

1. How did you feel when sharing your creation?

2. What are some of the ways you are different from the way others see you?

3. How accurately do you think you preceive yourself?

4. Do you feel good about the way others perceive you, about the way you perceive yourself?

Activity #2: Who's Who of the Week

Grade level: 5th grade

Materials needed: background information on students in class, construction paper, paste.

Background information: An emerging task in education today is to define selfesteem and to discover the process by which it is nurtured. The ultimate in selfesteem is found in the full possession of one's total being - the intellect and the emotions and (especially) the body - in other words, in the self.

Objective: To enhance student selfconcept using personal data and positive reinforcement of accomplishments.

Procedures:

1. Compile a "Who's Who Bulletin Board."

2. Data can be gathered about achievements, hobbies, pets, future goals, family members, etc.

3. Phone calls to students' homes may uncover information special to students while promoting health education to the parents.

4. When data is collected and written up, duplicate and distribute to all students in the class.

5. Pictures may accompany written information for a personal touch.

6. Designate one student per week to be recognized as "Who's Who Student of the Week."

7. Present bulletin board materials to honored student at end of the week.

Activity #3: Who Am I?

Grade level: 3rd grade

Materials needed: 3x5 notecards, pencils.

Background information: Every person needs recognition. It is expressed cogently by the lad who says, "Mother, let's play darts. I'll throw the darts and you say 'Wonderful.' " [3]

To enhance student selfconcept using students' own thoughts and ideas. To give the student recognition from teacher and classmates.

Procedure:

1. Have students write out biographical information. Include such things as talents, family happenings, hobbies, favorite places, activities, etc.

2. Collect the cards.

3. On occasion, read the cards at the beginning or end of class.

4. Include a teacher description also.

As health educators, promoting positive selfconcept in the classroom can be challenging but quite rewarding. By creatively letting loose, involving the students, giving students' recognition, and by allowing the student to *feel* in the classroom setting, a teacher can creatively enhance positive selfconcepts. As a kindergarten student put it, "When you ask me how I feel, I'm the only one who can tell you! And I like that!" [4]

[1]Vasconcellos, J., Chairman of the Joint Legislative Committee on Educational Goals and Evaluation, Member of the California Legislature.
[2]Purkey, W. W. *Self-concept and school achievement*. Englewood Cliffs, New Jersey: Prentice-Hall, Inc., 1970.
[3]Baughman, M. D. *Educator's handbook of stories, quotes, and humor*.
[4]Canfield, J., & Wells, H. C. *100 ways to enhance self-concept in the classroom*. Englewood Cliffs, New Jersey: Prentice-Hall, Inc., 1976, p. 207.

Ideas from a Class in Interpersonal Relations

CAROLL KAISER teaches health education at Minnetonka Senior High School, Excelsior, Minnesota. Her interpersonal relations classes, composed of sophomores, juniors, and seniors, are the most popular of the ten health classes offered for credit.

Interpersonal relations stresses the importance of self-image and self-acceptance in the development of personality. Without a secure self-image and a healthy self-acceptance, a person cannot risk the emotional investment necessary to relate to another individual. With a secure self-image and healthy self-acceptance, a person can risk the necessary emotional investment, and he gradually acquires a repertoire of successful behavior. Building this repertoire of successful behavior is a process of becoming and individuation. Thus, a cyclical evolvement takes place: self-image and self-acceptance determine the quality of interpersonal behavior; the quality of the interpersonal behavior determines the growth of personality; the growth of personality determines self-image and self-acceptance.

Some of the techniques I use in the interpersonal relations classes attempt to improve self-image and self-acceptance in order to develop a repertoire of successful interpersonal behavior. One device is what I call "Laws of the Robot." In this experiment I try to show students that the human condition is coped with, understandably and even justifiably, on a nonrational, even emotional, basis, and that this is not bad. In the Laws of the Robot, I pose hypothetical situations which students must try to solve using a purely computerized type of logic. My direction to students is that they

are to consider themselves as robots. Before they are allowed to enter human society, they must take a test to determine whether the "three laws" which are built into their robot being are functioning properly. The laws are a functional part of the circuitry and I further emphasize that all circuits are logical and cannot be altered in any way without serious damage, and that as robots they cannot violate the three laws either through action or through inaction. The laws are rigid, almost mechanical:

1. A robot may not injure a human or through inaction allow a human to come to harm.
2. A robot must obey orders given it by a human except where such an order might conflict with the first law.
3. A robot must protect its own existence as long as such protection does not conflict with the first or second law.

Before the exercise is over the students become bogged down and almost disfunctional in solving the hypothetical situations. To their great frustration, logic is not enough for a solution because nonlogical ramifications of the problem must be taken into account.

Another device I use for teaching self-awareness and self-acceptance is what I call the "Protoplasmic Blobs." These are a series of drawings or blobs faintly resembling humans, which elicit student interpretations of what the blobs are feeling. Since it is relatively easy to catalog gestures that people use to intensify statements, I felt that I could use protoplasmic blobs to illustrate the subtlety of gestures, the idea being that if a student could perceive the gestures in this experiment, he might more readily perceive them in his everyday living. Interpreting these characters is similar in a sense to the process people go through to interpret the Rorschach Ink Blot Test. This particular exercise is used in conjunction with a unit on body language. The exercise consists of 26 blob illustrations on a paper. At the bottom of the page are listed 26 comments. The students match each comment with the blob character it best expresses. For example, a student may interpret two characters as "quarreling," and he would supply a comment most appropriate for that depiction which might be, "please forgive me just one more time." Students can work individually or in a group where students compare their different interpretations. Incidentally, this exercise can lead to some interesting and effective role playing.

The "Environmental Box" idea is used toward the end of the unit on self-awareness as a final project. It is especially effective and rewarding for those students who are not adept verbally. The students are asked to portray or depict in visible form a concept or feeling they possess. They are to "remove" this feeling from environmental competition by "placing" it in a shoe box, fix the cover on the box, and then cut a hole in one end for the observer. Peering into the box and observing these visual manifestations of a student's inner life in complete isolation from an outside environmental force is a most cogent experience. The strength of this project lies in the fact that the completed assignment ranges from the most simple illustration to the most complex and intricate ones, involving, in some cases, mirrors, electric lights, and small models to create illusory effects.

Since communication is an integral part of interpersonal relations, I have used as an additional technique a short unit on the sign language of the deaf. Often, in the verbal language we use in everyday conversation, parallel conversations are conducted in which one person is not really listening to the other. Ultimately, after much parallel conversation, the art of real listening is lost. Teaching students basic sign language makes them aware for the first time of the intensity and the miracle of human communication. One is forced to look at and study the person who is doing the communicating. One sees all the nuances and connotations of what is said and felt. One of the high spots in this unit is a lecture given in sign language by a deaf lecturer. The intensity and concentration observed at this point is worth a whole year of teaching. I might add that teaching this skill is not difficult or time-consuming, and the hand alphabet can be learned in 15 or 20 minutes. Since there are hand gestures that make up entire words rather than spelling out each letter in the word, I also introduce five or ten hand gestures every day until each student develops quite an extensive vocabulary.

Role Playing as a Tool in Mental Health Education

Lynn Teper is assistant professor of health educa-tion at Long Island University, Brooklyn Center, Brooklyn, New York. She was formerly an in-structor at Kingsborough Community College in Brooklyn.

Teachers of health education must transmit to students the concept that physical and mental health are interrelated. Each is an aspect of the total individual; each is dependent on the other for optimal functioning. Formerly the mental component of health was overshadowed by health educators in their attempt to educate the student about bodily functions, but gradually, mental health has gained importance and is now a significant aspect of many health education cur-riculums. Through units in mental health, it is hoped that students will learn to meet with some adequacy their personal, interpersonal, and social conflicts and thus will function more completely as young adults.

One of the tools available for promoting healthy behavioral patterns is known as "socio-drama." Sociodrama is a spontaneous, impromptu expression dramatizing intergroup relations and collective ideologies. The students who play a role in a sociodrama do not recite from a script. A situation is presented to the class and without prior preparation students are chosen or volun-teer to act out the particular situation.

Man is a role player, in a sense, every day of his life. An adolescent girl, for example, can be a daughter, a friend, a student, a member of a club, etc. Each individual is characterized by a certain range of roles which dominates his or her behav-ior. The role player in a sociodrama is aware that he is acting out a role, even though he may be unaware that the role, as he enacts it, reveals many of the conflicts that confront him and others.

The process of sociodrama unfolds as follows:

Step 1—Sensitizing the group

It is important for the participants to recognize that people perceive and interpret situations and stimuli differently. As a result of their particular interpretation, attitudes are developed by each individual which result in different responses. This understanding can be gained by having sev-eral students view and report on a given situation. The result will usually yield a variety of opinions as to what took place, as when witnesses are asked to report on an accident or crime. This will reveal to some degree the lack of reliability be-tween observers due to a predisposition to select different aspects of the situation for notation. In addition, it will help students to see that their way of seeing and interpreting situations is not the only way.

Step 2—The Warm Up

This step involves setting up the situation for the sociodrama to take place. Topics for enact-ment can include conflict with the family, peer group relationships, attitudes involved with topics included in sex education or the use of narcotics. The instructor states the situation somewhat ab-stractly. Roles are described and volunteers are selected or chosen. For example: A girl is troubled by the fact that she is given little freedom from her parents. At this point someone is chosen for the role of the girl, another for the role of the mother; father and possibly a sister or brother can enter the scene.

Step 3—The Enactment

At this point, without any additional prepara-tion the role players act out what they believe would happen when the family was together.

Step 4—Helping the audience observe intelligently

Much of the value of sociodrama depends on the discussion with the class following the spon-taneous dramatization. Some of the questions could be:

1. Do you feel that the enactment was realistic?
2. As future parents, what do you believe the role of the parent should be?
3. How do you think parents and their children can come to better understand one another?

In other situations as well as this one the prime concern should be to discuss causes of behavior and appropriate ways of behaving and to encourage self-appraisal.

Step 5—Replaying the situation

It is helpful for students to see how the situation looks from different angles by switching roles. The daughter may become the parent or volunteers may replace those who have already participated. This will bring additional insights into the situation.

Step 6—The Evaluation

In the evaluation it is important to emphasize that with positive flexible attitudes individual growth takes place. Students need to discover for themselves that anxiety, fears, and immobility are not inherent in an object, event, or person, but are within themselves. The individual needs a positive attitude toward change. To say "I'll try" means motivation for growth is present.

If real learning is to take place, problems studied in school should deal with crucial situations in the lives of the student no matter what the subject area may be. The use of sociodrama in health education classes is one way to implement this approach since it allows students to explore some appropriate ways of dealing with others as well as with themselves. It is a process whereby one can look at familiar conflicts seen through the eyes of others. Subsequently, recognition that one is not alone in some of his confrontations may result in lessening anxiety. A three way process is established.

1. The teacher relates with the students through interest and involvement.

2. The students relate with one another by participating, observing, and commenting on the sociodrama.

3. The students relate to the teacher by referring to the teacher for guidance and structure.

Moralizing by the teacher is curbed and condemnation and judgment by an adult figure are eliminated.

Involvement is a key to understanding for students. Whether the student is a role player or part of the discussion group that evaluates the sociodrama, involvement is a significant outcome. Conflicts often will be left unresolved, but hopefully the students will have witnessed or have been a part of acting out and discussing a variety of ways for promoting healthy interactions involving the individual in his environment.

THE MIRROR GAME[1]

ROSA SULLIVAN is a health education teacher at Herbert Hoover Junior High, Lackawanna, New York 14218.

It is so extremely important for individuals to be able to look back on themselves in order to be evaluative of their personality traits. Many times people cannot detect their negative faults or, in contrast, tend only to find negative traits. A mentally healthy individual should be able to search on both sides and progress to working out "bad" traits. The following activity is one way to work toward this.

Objectives

1. To have a better understanding of who you are as you see yourself.
2. To have a better understanding of how others see you.
3. To recognize and understand that others always do not see you as you see yourself.
4. To appreciate the fact that you have negative points and evaluate how to change them if you wish to.
5. To evaluate how others see you and decide if that is your true image.

The Game

Duplicate a list of 20-30 personality traits suitable to the students' age group. (The group I used this game with was 14 years of age and enrolled at a junior high school.) Set them up in columns with room for graduated ratings of self and partner. (See example.)

Procedure

1. Have each student pick a partner with whom they are familiar.
2. After passing out the list, stress that they are not to talk while they are evaluating themselves or their partner.
3. The groups have 10-15 minutes to make their judgments.

4. They then compare what they marked about themselves and each other. This should reveal a number of differences between their self-impressions and how they are perceived by others. This may take as long as 15-20 minutes.
5. During the last 5 minutes in class and continued as a home assignment, students should write on the back of their papers three things they learned

about themselves that they did not know before. They should also explain what these three things mean to them.

Follow up

(15-20 minutes of another class or as a home assignment)

1. With your class go over the list and mark each word as either positive or negative (example: if you marked always or sometimes for sensitive then it is positive; if you marked seldom or never for sensitive then it is negative).
2. A sheet containing the following questions is then passed out and the teacher requests the student to be as truthful as possible in responding since no one will see their answers without their expressed permission.

   What image did you project to your partner?

   What are some of the traits you feel you possess but others do not feel you possess?

   Why do your perceptions differ from others' perceptions?

   Do you have a strong self-image? (Do you like yourself or if you weren't you, would you like you?)

   Do you have more negative or **positive traits? Why?**

   Everyone has traits they do not like. Think about two of your negative ones and explain how you can go about changing them.

[1] Adapted from *Go To Health* (New York: Dell Publishing Co., Inc., 1972), p. 98.

TRAITS		SELF				PARTNER			
		Never	Seldom	Sometimes	Always	Never	Seldom	Sometimes	Always
1. Sensitive	+								
2. Arrogant	−								
3. Silly	−								
4. Trusting	+								
5. Tender	+								
6. Two-faced	−								

How to Cope with Stress in the Classroom

CHARLES C. DAVIS is coordinator for health/physical education instructional programs, State University College at Oswego, Oswego, New York 13126.

Learning alternatives for handling stressful situations and then giving students an experience in handling stress and developing coping ability is something often left out of the classroom. As educators we often find it difficult to place students in situations where they can learn practically how to handle various stressors. Much of what we say is abstract or theoretical until the student is forced to confront stress. The following stress sheet is designed as a practical way for students to identify stress and then analyze how they cope with various stressful situations. A deeper discussion of stress and the learning of alternative situations to various life problems can be better understood. The stress sheet is adaptable for many age groups and grade levels.

Step 1: Content

The students are taught the intricate details of life and stress in their class. The following aspects are reviewed.

1. The stress concept—what is stress? discussion of Hans Selyé's theory of stress.
2. Stress as it affects our lives—stress is not inherently good or evil, it is dependent on the consequences of our reactions to stressors.
3. Coping with stress—General Adaptation Syndrome (GAS), the physiological response to stress; flight/flee response or coping behavior (general alternatives).
4. Learning ways to cope with stress—protecting the ego ideal under stressful situations; defense mechanisms; Maslow's hierarchy of human needs.
5. Adapting to stress—suggestions for learning to cope with stress in a constructive manner; positive and negative consequences of deviations.

Step 2: Learning to Cope with Stress Constructively

Students are given a stress sheet to relate classroom theory to actual confrontations with stressful situations. The students are asked to take the following stress sheet home and fill it out after undergoing stress.

Stress Sheet

This sheet is designed to stimulate interest in and an understanding of how you react to and cope with stress. It is also hoped that completion of this sheet will cause you to do some reflective thinking on how to handle the "wear and tear of life" or stress.

1. Identify: A stressful situation; the stressor(s), internal and/or external primary stimulus causing the stress.

2. Which of the following behavioral responses did you use to cope with the stress? Place an x next to how you responded.
   Fight   Freeze   Flight
          Compromise
   Briefly describe the consequences of your response: it did _____ did not _____ alleviate the stressful situation.

3. Check any defense mechanisms that you used to deviate from the stressor.
   _____ avoidance _____ regression
   _____ deny reality
   _____ fixation
   _____ repression _____ sublimation
   _____ projection
   _____ other (specify)
   _____ rationalization

4. Draw a line to indicate how you expended energy as you progressed through the Adaptation Syndrome.

5. Sources of help. Did talking with anyone help you cope with or adapt to the stressor?
no _____ yes _____
specify whom _____

6. What deviations did you use to equalize the effect of the stress on the body? (for example sports, reading, etc., please specify). Briefly describe how your deviations relieved the stress.

7. Did any psychologically induced pain cause a physical reaction?
no _____ yes _____
specify _____ e.g., prolonged tension leads to upset stomach.

Step 3: Behavioral Outcomes

After taking home a predetermined number of stress sheets the students should have some stress-relieving skills, such as the following.

1. Analyze some of the stressors common to the experiences of students, such as competition or failure.

2. Understand the meaning of the terms stress, stressors, stressful situations.

3. Analyze the individual use of defense mechanisms in stressful situations used to minimize conscious anxiety.

4. Understand that humans are affected by and respond to stressors as total organisms.

5. Understand the general categories of behavioral responses to stress: flight, fight or compromise.

6. Understand the consequences of conversion reactions such as psychologically induced pain manifesting physical reactions when stressors are not successfully adapted to or deviated from.

7. Investigate how individual coping behaviors (sports, dancing, etc.) successfully allow an individual to alleviate stressors.

Step 4: Classroom Adaptability

1. Students can be asked to do several stress sheets over an extended period, then analyze how they cope with and adapt to stress.

2. Break students into small discussion groups, give each group the job of depicting: what is stress? or what is mental health? or what is the relationship between stress and mental health?

Give each group about 20 minutes to come up with their pictorial descriptions. No words can be used in any of the three assignments. When the allotted time has ended, the instructor holds up the finished product from one group and the class responds to what they see depicted. The same is done for the other groups. The instructor phrases the questions in a way which will extract the relationship between stress and mental health.

The outcome of the stress sheets exercise encompasses the interrelationship of the theory of stress and how it relates to mental health by personalizing stress through the stress sheets and visually depicting the wide interpretations of what stress is.

Mental Health

Coping With Violence

ELAINE HALS teaches at the South Shore High School in Brooklyn, New York 11236.

What can we as health educators do to reverse or at least slow down the chain of violence with which our students live? Our objectives should be: (1) to have students consider *all* life as positive, (2) to guide students in establishing constructive goals for the future, (3) to help students explore their values and priorities, (4) to help students explore the impact of violence on our society, and (5) to assist students in finding nonviolent methods of handling potentially explosive situations.

These are difficult objectives to reach. How do we achieve them? One way is to plan for the mental health segment of the required health course (or any other appropriate segment, e.g., urban problems, crime, values and goals) to include discussion topics and activities such as the following.

Topics

1. Prejudice—its causes and relationship to violence
2. Respect for the views of others
3. Respect for the property of others
4. Peer pressure; gang involvement
5. Values formation (clarification); priorities
6. Constructive methods of problem solving and dealing with stress
7. Setting realistic goals for the future
8. The impact of violence on our society
   Fear of involvement
   Fear of going out alone
   Tendency to overreact
   Crimes committed in self-defense
   People arming themselves
   Acceptance of violent deaths as statistics
9. Need for feelings of self-esteem
   Being recognized by others as worthwhile
10. Constructively compensating for weaknesses
11. Handling emotions—learning to think before acting
12. Working towards a healthier society
    How?
    Role of the individual
13. Value of life—own and others
    Everyone is important to someone

Activities

1. Role playing
   Mock court case
   Student caught cheating
   Racial or ethnic role reversals
2. Values activity
   Have students rate the following as acceptable or unacceptable for themselves. Discuss reasons for each student's choice.
   a. breaking laws they don't believe in
   b. law enforcement agencies
   c. smoking marijuana
   d. our government
   e. cheating
   f. demonstrations against the establishment
   g. compare students' values with those of their parents
   h. capital punishment
   i. plea bargaining
3. *Search for Values* (Pfaum/Standard, Cincinnati, Ohio 1974). Read section on Time, Lesson 3: "Examining Personal Goals"
4. Simon, Sidney B., Howe, L. W., Kirschenbaum, Howard, *Values Clarification: A Handbook of Practical Strategies for Teachers and Students* (Hart Pub. Co., New York, 1974). Play the Bomb Shelter Game (prejudice) and the Transplant Game.

5. Am I Worthwhile Task
   Have each student talk about self for two minutes saying *only* good things. Do this activity in groups. Have the group members help the individual speaking whenever necessary. The purpose of this activity is to help each student see that he or she is worthwhile.
6. Values Auction from *Auction Game* by Richard Cohen in his graduate course, "Health Education in the Secondary Schools," at Brooklyn College.
   Give each student an imaginary $1,-000 to bid with, give them a values list, and hold an auction. If several students are willing to bid the entire $1,000, have each give his or her reason for wanting the item and then allow the class to vote. After the auction evaluate student priorities.

Items To Be Auctioned

1. Invitations to all the most exciting parties (any place with anyone in the whole world) every single night.
2. To possess perfect health and a strong, flexible, beautiful, graceful body.
3. A lifetime without "hassling." No one will tell you what to do or how or when to do it.
4. A daily "storm" of new ideas; original poems, songs, books, movies running through your head; visions of paintings to paint, pots to mold, buildings to design and build.
5. To be the richest person in the world.
6. The opportunity to direct the workings of the whole world . . . to control individuals, businesses, monies, whole nations.
7. No "hang-ups" whatsoever; to possess self-knowledge.
8. A chance to spend a year with the greatest religious figure of your faith—past, present, future.
9. To live forever without growing old.
10. The opportunity to stick up for and protect the person or thing to which you feel the greatest allegiance (like sticking with a friend through a crisis or fighting for your country, etc.).
11. To have the perfect romance/or the perfect love relationship (s) with the person (s) of your choice.
12. To have a computer-bank of facts and information in your head; to be able to answer any questions and solve any problems which present themselves to you.
13. To have the strength always to do what you believe to be right. To be a person of integrity.
14. To have the skills, know-how, and time to really help others and serve humanity.
15. To have a real sense of what is fair and just; to deal with others as honestly and fairly as possible.
16. To be at peace with yourself and know the purpose of life.
17. To become a professional athlete of your choice.

Health educators will not be able to eliminate violence, but we can encourage our students to examine the causes and end results of violence. We can show them more constructive outlets for their anger and their frustrations, as well as how to set and reach positive goals for the future.

Personality Spokes

ROSA SULLIVAN is a health education teacher at Herbert Hoover Junior High School, Lackawanna, New York 14218.

Man has qualities about himself that are of great value to him in reference to future ambitions. He also has faults and because of these he sometimes is incapable of accomplishing goals. It is a necessary objective of life to be able to recognize both faults and positive attributes which can hinder or enhance man in his quest of the future.

At what age should a person begin to examine his own personality to establish priorities in life and plans to achieve in these areas? The answer is it is never too soon to initiate at home or in the classroom, activities to stimulate thinking in these areas. Personality Spokes is one activity to achieve this end.

Objectives

For students to—

1. Recognize assets in their personalities.

2. Recognize faults in their personalities.

3. Delve into themselves and be able to establish short and long-term goals.

4. Evaluate what faults and assets will help them to achieve or fail to reach their goals.

5. Communicate with others what they find out about themselves.

Procedure

1. Have each student pick a partner.

2. Each student is to draw three half dollar size circles: two at

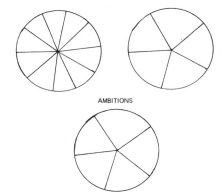

the top and one at the bottom of a piece of paper (see example). Next he is to draw spokes as if these circles were wheels. One top circle has 10 spokes and is labeled personality assets. The other top circle has 5 spokes and is labeled faults. The bottom wheel has 5 spokes and is labeled ambitions.

3. Each student is to fill in the spokes accordingly, examine what they wrote and then draw lines from the assets to the ambitions these assets will help satisfy. Then the student is to draw lines from the faults to the ambitions that these faults will prevent from satisfying.

4. The students should then exchange and examine each other's papers.

5. Each student next explains to partner why these assets and faults will help or hinder his ambitions. They also should talk about *how* important these ambitions are to them, and *why* they are so important.

Mental Health

About Yourself

RUTH C. ENGS is assistant professor, Department of Health and Safety Education, Indiana University, Bloomington, Indiana 47401.

A "mentally healthy" person is often characterized as having an accurate perception of reality, able to maintain close interpersonal relationships, able to communicate openly and honestly with others, and aware of personal goals, values, abilities, and behavior.[1] Because of the variety of environmental stresses and our individual backgrounds, we all have different problems of living. The extent to which we learn to successfully cope with these stresses often determines how mentally healthy we are.

One of the primary objectives of mental health education in the classroom is to help the student become aware of himself, his communication techniques, and his behavior as an aid in learning to cope successfully with life. The following warm up can help the student become acquainted with himself, with others, and

with the class as a whole. It can help to create an atmosphere for fostering open communication and self-knowledge leading to better mental health.

These instructions should be related to the class by the instructor:

We are now going to do some get acquainted exercises. We first will do a relaxation exercise to tune in to ourselves. Then we will do several exercises to get to know others in the class. This may be a new experience for some of you, however, most people find it fun. If for some reason you find you do not wish to continue, you can stop at any time. However, I'm sure you will find it enjoyable.

Relaxation (10 minutes)

1. First put your head on your desk and get comfortable in your chair or lie down on the floor and get comfortable.
2. Close your eyes, relax, and become aware of the sounds in the room.
3. Next, I want you to pay attention to your breathing. Feel the air go in and out.
4. Now I want you to take a deep breath, feel the air going in your lips, down into your lungs; feel air go out. (Repeat this two times.)
5. You should feel relaxed; in fact, it is probably the first time you have relaxed today.
6. Now become aware of your feet, feel them against the floor, in your shoes. Now tighten your feet as long as you can. Now relax.
7. Become aware of your calf, (continue with thighs, whole leg, shoulder and buttocks, chest, fist, neck, face, whole body).
8. You will feel relaxed; become aware of parts of your body, touching the chair (floor).
9. Now relax. And take a deep breath.

Body Trip[2]—The Magic Golden Ball (10 minutes)

To be used after people are in a relaxed state.

Imagine that you see a warm golden ball in front of you.

As you watch it, it slowly begins to shrink becoming smaller and smaller.

When it is the size of a dime it moves toward you.

It gets closer and closer and finally attaches to your forehead.

Then it turns into a magic warm golden paint.

It flows over your forehead, nose. Smell it, taste it.

As it flows it feels warm and glowing.

When it reaches your neck the magical paint takes on different colors and still flows over your body—shoulders, upper arms, lower arms, fingers, chest,

stomach, genetalia, thighs, legs, feet, toes.

You are now surrounded in a warm bath of colors and feel good. I will count backward from 10 to 1. While I am counting, start opening your eyes. At the count of 1 you will be wide awake and feel good.

I now want you to turn to the person next to you and discuss what you experienced.

Getting Acquainted[3]

1. Go up to someone you do not know but think you might have something in common with and would like to know better. One person talks for two minutes while the other just listens. Then reverse the role. Now, the two of you find another pair you do not know. Introduce your partner to the other pair.
2. Go up to someone you think you have nothing in common with. Sit back to back and talk. Join another pair and discuss things you learned about communication by sitting back to back.
3. Go up to another person you do not know. Look each other in the eyes. Do not talk. Follow each other's hands around as if you were looking in a mirror. Join another pair and discuss what you learned about yourself and the other person by doing this.

Debriefing

1. Get back into a big circle. What did you experience with the fantasy trip?
2. How does it feel to go up to a stranger and talk?
3. How much did you find you had in common with the person you thought you had nothing in common with?
4. What problems did you have in communicating back to back?
5. What did you learn about nonverbal communication or about your own communication skills from sitting back to back?
6. Who led in the hand mirroring? Why? What did you learn about yourself in this exercise, about the other person?

[1] Maslow, Abraham H., *Toward A Psychology of Being*, 2nd edition, Van Nostrand-Reinholt Co., Toronto, 1968.

[2] Adopted from Dick Price's "Gestalt Workshop," Esalen Institute, Big Sur, California.

[3] Pfeiffer, J., and Jones, J., *A Handbook of Structured Experiences for Human Relations Training*, Vol. I-IV, University Associates, Iowa City, Iowa.

A Lesson on Stress

JANET H. SHIRREFFS is in the Department of Physiology and Health Science, Ball State University, Muncie, Indiana 47306.

A generally accepted educational principle is that students learn best in an environment in which certain moderate to high expectations are made clear to students but is only minimally or moderately stressful. Excessive stress may be so incapacitating that no effort on the part of the individual can alleviate it. It is impossible for learning to take place in an overly stressful environment in which the adaptive potential of students is exceeded. Of course, individuals differ in both perceptions of stress and in their ability to cope with stress and conflict in their daily lives and these differences are important considerations for the educator in discussing stress and emotional health.

Although health educators cannot teach mental health *per se*, it is possible to provide classroom experiences dealing with mental health and the solution of every day problems which can help students tune-in to real life situations, feel the emotions they evoke, and analyze actions and behaviors which

they can use to alleviate these emotional crises in constructive, appropriate ways. This is the case in the following classroom technique:

Goal: (1) Learn what stress is
(2) Learn what anxiety and/or anger feels like as the result of encountering a stressful experience
(3) Learn how stress can best be handled in positive and constructive ways to resolve problems and reduce feelings of being "overwhelmed" by appropriate individual action.

Level: This classroom experience has been used effectively at the college level during a unit on mental health. The learning experience would also be applicable at the senior and junior high school level with some modification.

Method: (1) Students should be fairly comfortable with teacher and vice-versa.
(2) Class environment should be humanistic and typically low-stress prior to the experience.
(3) Teacher should have made evaluation requirements of the class very specific, including an announcement that no unannounced quizzes would be given during the semester.

Following introductory class periods devoted to personality development and enhancement of mental health, the instructor should enter class with a test or quiz which has been prepared from materials the students were supposed to have read and additional questions which are not from the assigned readings. Below is an example of a test of this type.

HES 100 Personal Health
Quiz 1
Emotional Health

1. List Erikson's Eight States of Personality Development. (8 points)
2. In defining and describing the psychotic personality disorders, the text speaks of organic and functional causes. Describe each. (4 points)
3. Give three examples of character disorders. (3 points)
4. According to the text, what is anxiety? (5 points)

Keeping very serious, announce: "You will be having a test now, please remove all materials from your desks." You will notice abrupt changes in facial expression, body movements etc., ranging from panic to anger which can provide a basis for a discussion of bodily manifestations of anxiety.

Pass out tests. Allow the students about three minutes to look over the test and announce: "Write your feelings at this moment on the bottom of the test paper." A number of reactions actual students have reported during this activity are: complete confusion; helpless; I would like to throw my chair at you for springing this on me; anger; complete nothingness; a burst of adrenalin shot through my system; disgust and frustration; my heart fell, anxiety, shocked, confused; feeling of total lack of control; insecure; I am feeling completely lost and kind of scared.

Announce immediately after you have asked the students to record their feelings on the bottom of the test page: "This is not a real test, but an experience to get each of you to realize right now what stressful situations can make you feel like inside. (You will hear sighs of relief, laughter, and comments such as "I didn't think you'd do anything like this to us, whew!")

STRESS MODEL

| | **Stress** | | |
| Anxiety | Frustration | Anger | **Emotional Responses** |

Endocrine functioning as a consequence of parasympathetic system's reactions to stress

| | **Stress** | | |
| Adrenalin | | Non-adrenalin | **Physiological Response** |

Increase in blood pressure. heart rate, sweating, dilation of pupils, etc.

| *Flight* | *Fight* | *Internalization with no release* | **Behavioral Adaptation** |

Individual differences in alleviating stress

Potentially constructive

Deal with anxiety and anger as they occur in small pieces.

Be assertive, honest, and real when situations involving people create feelings of anxiety or anger.

Select and use appropriate physical outlets for venting anger and anxiety (running, cycling, playing tennis, or playing piano).

Appropriate use of defense mechanisms.

Potentially destructive

Let anger and anxiety build up by not recognizing internal feelings and/or by not acting on them.

Be aggressive and outwardly hostile or submissive when situations involving people create feelings of anxiety or anger.

Attempt to hold in and repress feelings of anger and anxiety and try to forget the situations that caused them.

Inappropriate overuse of defense mechanisms.

Discussion: General questions which relate to this experience include: What is stress? What situations are stressful to you? How can stress resulting in anger or anxiety be handled constructively and destructively? What do you do with anger when you feel it? What are some constructive outlets for anger and anxiety? What do you think are the dangers of repressed anger and anxiety?

Lecture: The model presented on the next page can serve as a framework for a lecture on stress, including its emotional, physiological, and behavioral parameters. Health-generating resolution of stress should be emphasized.

Health educators cannot eliminate the many stresses their students will encounter in their daily lives. They can, however, help students to examine the types of situations which evoke individual stress reactions and can discuss alternative ways of coping with stress, so that young people will be able to incorporate health-generating behaviors into stress-provoking situations in their lifestyles.

Mental Health Auctioning Strategy

PATRICK KIDD TOW is an assistant professor in the Department of Health and Physical Education at Old Dominion University, Norfolk, Virginia 23508.

This teaching strategy is appropriate for secondary school or college level health classes. I have used it at the end of a mental health or drug education unit, but it might also be applicable to any health unit which uses value clarification.

Each participant begins with a set sum of money—let us say $25,000, and is entrusted to keep a running tally of how much they have spent and what was bought. Members of the class bid on certain aspirations, loves, or wishes in an auction. The items for auction could pertain to physical, emotional, social, or even spiritual health.

The instructor plays the part of an auctioneer. Only he or she should know what items are up for auction and should try to keep the bids as high as possible. Fervor and interest will grow as the soaring bids become more competitive. The auctioneer should deal with each item one at a time by announcing and writing it on the board. After the final bid is accepted, the selling price is written next to the item.

The objective of this strategy is to evoke introspection on what values the individual cherishes. At the same time, students can see which behaviors and values are held in high esteem by their peers. The impulsive and eccentric nature of some participants may also become apparent. After completing the exercise, there will soon be an influx of comments and questions from the results.

The following items have been auctioned off in a mental health class.

1. Guarantee to die a peaceful and painless death when the time comes
2. Ability to prevent World War III
3. Ten extra years added on to your life
4. Never have to work and still be paid
5. Ability to save the life of one person
6. Phenomenal love for children
7. Ability to play any musical instrument desired
8. Be boss and sole owner of a company
9. Own the only solar-powered sports car

10. Travel back or forward in time and change history
11. Be considered a fantastic lover
12. Be the most loved and popular politician in the country
13. Never have a sick day in your life
14. Possess unrivaled intelligence or genius
15. Eat as much as you want and never get fat
16. Be the author of the world's best-selling book
17. Be considered a successful financial wizard
18. Be exceptionally skilled in any sports one desires
19. Phenomenal love for animals
20. Never have an enemy in the world, be loved by all
21. Die with a clean conscience, no debts, and no sins left behind
22. Guarantee to never become addicted to any drugs
23. Climb the highest mountain and survive

24. Be granted more handsomeness or beauty
25. Reincarnation into anything or anyone desired

Additional objectives may be achieved by modifying this auctioning strategy. Following are some suggestions.

Reduce or increase the number of items to suit a specific health topic being covered.

Distribute a list of items for auction so they may be arranged according to individual preferences.

Allow small groups to submit public bids as a consensus.

Permit borrowing or lending of money among participants to see how many overextend themselves.

People Labeling Strategy

PATRICK K. TOW and HAL WINGARD are assistant professors in the Department of Health and Physical Education at Old Dominion University, Norfolk, Virginia 23508.

Categories of People

Labels	parent	teacher	neighbor	TV star	stranger	Total
Alcoholic						
Mentally Disturbed						
Homosexual						
Drug Addict						
Divorcee						
Total						

Many people are in the habit of labeling or stereotyping other members of society. Some of these "tagged victims" may be acquaintances of those doing the labeling. While peer group coercion has been able to provide the necessary motivation for constructive changes in our lives, it can also be destructive in nature. The insidious manner in which labels and stories can spread help blow the picture far out of proportion. Perhaps someday we may come to realize such practices tend to do more harm than good.

An innocent person defamed by a circulating, malicious slander may feel the intense social and emotional impacts. Public denial of such labels may be interpreted as frantic attempts to conceal guilt. There is always that tragic alternative of the stigmatized acting in accordance with the label bestowed upon him. On the other hand, there is also the possibility that a label accurately depicts a person's past or present. Nevertheless, such unscrupulous denotations expressed out of spite or ignorance tend to diminish the faith and trust one has in one's fellow man.

Stigmatization is only one part of the concern. The other is one which many of us fall prey to on a number of occasions. Our fear surfaces when listening ears begin to believe and treat a person according to that real or unreal stigma. Such occurrences may appear to be a concerted effort to prevent an individual from joining the mainstream of American society. Perhaps some people believe whatever actions are associated with a given label warrant public denouncement ad infinitum. The resulting social and emotional damages could be avoided if we were sensitized to the ramifications of our persistent "pigeonholing" behavior.

This teaching strategy is intended to draw out various prejudices, biases, and fears governing our lives. It will become obvious in discussions among high school or college students that some concerns are groundless and based upon sheer ignorance. However, there will be some thoughts expressed which were based on feelings derived from personal experiences which might not necessarily be refuted. Therefore, it becomes absolutely essential for teachers and students alike to pay heed to what is being said.

The teaching instrument to be used is shown as a table. The rows represent five types of labels apt to be used as brands for certain undesirables. The columns represent five categories of people that are hypothetically given the labels. Students are directed to correlate each label with every category of people and assign a score to indicate the degree of tolerability they have toward these individuals. The range of scores is: 4–will always be able to tolerate; 3–will frequently be able to tolerate; 2–will sometimes be able to tolerate; 1–will seldom be able to tolerate; 0–will never be able to tolerate.

Examples of the process involved should be provided for the students. For example, a student examines the hypothetical situation that one of his parents is an alcoholic. He may find that fact absolutely intolerable and assigns a score of zero. On the other hand, he may be quite willing most of the time to accept the fact that his favorite TV star turned out to be an alcoholic. If this is the case, the student would assign a score of three. In another example, a student may be willing to tolerate his homosexual teacher most of the time and scores a three. However, he may seldom feel tolerant enough to associate with a homosexual stranger and assigns a score of two.

A sum of totals from each row and column reflect that label or category of people deserving the most and least degree of tolerance. For example, the highest row total found associated with divorcee would suggest that student is more tolerant of divorcees than any of the other given labels. By the same token, the highest column total, which is associated with stranger, may indicate that student is more tolerant of their improprieties than the other category of people. The lowest row or column totals may indicate that label or category of people least tolerated by the student.

Other variables besides what is given in the table can be used in substitution. Any of the following can be added to people categories: brother/sister, politician, cousin, boy/girlfriend, or minister. Any of the following labels can be used, too: transsexual, shoplifter, murderer, marijuana smoker, hit-run driver, suicide attempter, child abuser, or bisexual. Of course, there are also other possible alternatives that can be conjured up by the teacher.

In the ensuing discussions, students should begin to realize people with such labels used in this strategy need more empathy than sympathy from other people. Most anyone can provide pity, but understanding is a step beyond what the stigmatized may expect. It is fortunate that changing times and people in today's world beckon us to relent and modify our opinions about others now deemed out of place in our society.

Nutrition

Creative Food Labels: Consumer Health Education

MOON S. CHEN, JR. *is visiting assistant professor, Department of Health, Physical Education, and Recreation, Box 4070, Texas Tech University, Lubbock, Texas 79409.*

Any unit or course in consumer health should include a section on what to expect on food labels. Described in the following outline is one way to facilitate student learning in food labels.

Teacher Preparation

1. Read the handout, "A Consumer's Guide to Food Labels," by Margaret Morrison from the June 1977 *FDA Consumer*.
2. Prepare enough copies of the handout for distribution to each student.
3. Write the names of approximately five to seven fresh fruits on strips of paper so that there are enough for each class member and each fruit is more or less equally represented.

Place these strips of paper in a bag. Students will draw these strips for their assignment.

Behavioral Expectations for the Student

As a result of this exercise, the student will be able to:

1. Make a food label and in doing so will be familiar with the various components of food labeling.
2. Make judgments on the quality of various food labels.
3. Experience, discuss, and categorize the decision-making processes of many consumers.

Procedure

Day One

1. Introduce the topic of food labeling with emphasis on reasons for labeling

food, FDA requirements for food labels, explanations of the various components of the nutrition information label.
2. Introduce the idea of a contest to be conducted the next class day on food labels. Each class member draws from a paper bag a choice of a fresh fruit. These choices are not to be revealed to other members of the class. For the next class assign students to read the handout, "A Consumer's Guide to Food Labels," and make a label for the choice they drew from the paper bag that would conform to FDA

guidelines. Any information that is not available, such as net weight, may be estimated or made up.

3. Announce that there will be prizes (first prize and runner-up) awarded to the most original label, the most popular label, the most attractive label.

Day Two

1. Have all those with the same fruits place their labels in one area of the classroom. The objective is to place labels in such a way that they will "sell" themselves. Have students put a price on their items.
2. Once labels are in place, distribute three pieces of paper to each student for ballots.
3. Instruct students to write their choices for the best label on their ballots. Students may distribute their voting on these ballots in any fashion they wish—all three ballots for their choice of best label, two ballots for one choice and one ballot for another, or one ballot for three different choices.

4. Invite volunteers to tally the ballots.
5. After the ballots have been tallied, announce the winning labels and award the prizes for the best label and runner-up. The teacher may decide what to do in case there are ties.
6. Prizes could be books or fruits.
7. The teacher should then follow up this exercise with a discussion on consumer decision-making in the marketplace and ask class to share their experiences and their decision-making.

Sensible Dieting

1. Investigate commercial health spas and community recreational facilities. Compare cost, services offered, equipment available, and reputation. Investigate commercial diet clinics comparing type and length of "treatment," promises made, food plan, consideration for changing food habits, and success rate.

MARILYN MUDGETT is associated with the Health Education Department, Group Health Cooperative. DOROTHY CULJAT is presently evaluating the weight control program of Group Health Cooperative, 200 15th Avenue East, Seattle, Washington 98112.

2. Make a study of doctors who specialize in weight control. Examine professional qualifications, length of treatment, types of treatments (pre-packaged foods, pills, shots, hypnosis, etc.), success rate, and possible health dangers.

Dieting is an obsession for many Americans. Money readily spent on fad diets, exercise devices, over-the-counter weight loss aids; miracle foods, and national self-help organizations all add up to a billion dollar weight reduction industry. Physical activity has been taken out of the realm of the natural and is under the domain of big business—health spas, athletic clubs.

The search to be thin can be confusing and costly to the consumer. Students need accurate, unbiased information to make decisions about weight control and learn how to protect their pocketbooks at the same time. The following assignments are methods of educating the potential consumer.

3. Visit the local drugstore and make a list of the over-the-counter reducing aids available or visit a library or bookstore and note the number and titles of books on dieting.

4. Compile magazine and newspaper advertisements on diets, diet aids, and slimming devices. Evaluate the reliability of these advertisements analyzing the use of objective facts, pseudoscientific words such as "cellulite" and "diuretic," or claims to do something for nothing such as, "lose ugly fat while you eat the foods you love."

5. Write to adolescent summer weight camps and adult "fat farms" for brochures. Figuring length of stay and desired weight to be lost, determine how much each pound of weight loss would cost.

6. Make a survey of family and friends to determine if they ever dieted, types of diets, aids, products and/or facilities used, success rate, and cost.

Two excellent resources for consumer education and weight control are *Thin From Within* by Jack Osman and *A Diet for Living* by Jean Mayer.